WHEN PARENTS DIE

Learning to live with the loss of a parent

Third edition

Rebecca Abrams

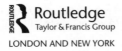
Routledge
Taylor & Francis Group

LONDON AND NEW YORK

First edition published 1992
by Charles Letts & Co. Ltd
Second edition published 1999
by Routledge
This edition published 2013
by Routledge
2 Park Square, Milton Park, Abingdon, Oxon, OX14 4RN

Simultaneously published in the USA and Canada
by Routledge
711 Third Avenue, New York, NY 10017

Routledge is an imprint of the Taylor & Francis Group, an informa business

© 2013 1999 1992 Rebecca Abrams

The right of Rebecca Abrams to be identified as author of this work has been asserted by her in accordance with sections 77 and 78 of the Copyright, Designs and Patents Act 1988.

British Library Cataloguing in Publication Data
A catalogue record for this book is available from the British Library

Library of Congress Cataloging-in-Publication Data
Abrams, Rebecca.
When parents die : learning to live with the loss of a parent /
Rebecca Abrams. -- 3rd ed.
p. cm.
1. Grief. 2. Bereavement--Psychological aspects. 3. Parents--Death--Psychological aspects. 4. Loss (Psychology) I. Title.
BF575.G7A25 2013
155.9'37--dc23
2012025038

ISBN13: 978-0-415-59011-2 (hbk)
ISBN13: 978-0-415-59012-9 (pbk)
ISBN13: 978-0-203-08101-3 (ebk)

Typeset in Baskerville
by Taylor & Francis Books

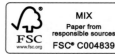

Printed and bound in Great Britain by
TJ International Ltd, Padstow, Cornwall

WHEN PARENTS DIE

The death of a parent marks an emotional and psychological watershed in a person's life. For children and teenagers the loss of a parent, if not handled sensitively, can be a lasting trauma, and for adults too a parent's death can be a tremendous blow.

When Parents Die speaks to bereaved children of all ages. Rebecca Abrams draws on her personal and professional knowledge of parental loss, as well as the experiences of many other adults, teenagers and children, to provide the reader with an honest, compassionate and insightful exploration of the experience of losing a parent. The book covers the entire course of grieving, from the period leading up to a parent's death through to recovery, paying particular attention to the many circumstances that can prolong and complicate mourning.

An indispensable aid to the bereaved, their families and the many professionals who work with them, this book is written in a clear and sympathetic style. It has been fully revised for this third edition to take into account recent research and new developments and understanding in the field of bereavement.

Rebecca Abrams is an award-winning author of both fiction and non-fiction. She worked as a bereavement counsellor for Cruse Bereavement Care and at the Cheltenham Ladies' College for a number of years, and regularly lectures and leads workshops on young people and parental bereavement. She is a tutor in creative writing at the University of Oxford and writer-in-residence at Larkmead School, Abingdon.

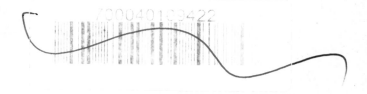

LETTERS FROM READERS

'At the age of 16 my life was devastated when my father committed suicide. The person who was so loving and vital a part of my life left a wife and daughter totally stunned, shocked, distraught ... I can't find the words to explain the feelings. This letter is to thank you for finally giving me the chance to realise that I'm not the only person who has felt this way. No professional has helped me as much. You have no idea how relieved I have been reading your book, and I thank you from the bottom of my heart for your warming and calming words. They have given me the strength to face and assess my father's death, and you have truly inspired me in my outlook on life and death.' Mary, aged 17

'Your book has been an enormous help to me and my family. It is the most realistic book currently on the market.' Julia, aged 27

'I only wish there had been a book like this available when my mother died when I was 18. As I read your book I kept saying, "Oh yes!" to myself as you clearly and honestly tackled so many familiar themes that have been part of my life.' Elizabeth, aged 43

'When I was 15, my stepfather died of cancer and less than two months later my mother committed suicide. Although this happened nearly four years ago, I am still hurting inside so much. Thank you for writing a book that addresses bereavement so well and truthfully. It has been so reassuring to learn that other people do undergo similar emotions after a bereavement. I've never read anything that puts my feelings so perfectly into words.' Jo, aged 19

'I have just finished reading your book and felt I had to tell you how profoundly moving and wonderful I think it is. I wish everyone whose parent dies could have this book.' Rachel, aged 23

'My mother died in November and it was her death that prompted me to buy your book a few days later. I came across it in a bookshop a few days before her funeral, opened it to see if it might be helpful, and knew I had to buy it. Thank you so much! Your book

has been a great comfort to me and I'm sure it will remain so for some time to come.' Pat, aged 44

'I first read When Parents Die *soon after my mum died, 14 years ago. Since then, I have often referred back to it when I've felt low or confused. The greatest message I took from this book is that everyone deals with grief differently, yet so many issues are covered in depth that it can help anyone going through the process.'* Richard, aged 29

'My mum died 13 years ago when I was 20. You wouldn't believe how much of a relief it is even after all these years to have the chaos and the fear I felt back then acknowledged at last, to have it recognised what a burden and unrealistic expectation is placed on the young person when people tell you you'll be fine, you can cope. You expressed my experience so vividly I was crying and saying out loud as I read, yes, yes, someone else knows and understands how it was.' Eluned, aged 33

TO THE MEMORY OF MY FATHER
AND MY STEPFATHER

CONTENTS

ACKNOWLEDGEMENTS

In the course of writing this book I have drawn on the ideas, memories, advice and support of a great many people. Some were professionals who kindly shared their knowledge and expertise with me, others were ordinary people brave enough to share their own painful memories and experiences. Deserving of special mention are Sarah Miller, who helped set up the self-help group at Cambridge that indirectly led to the first edition of this book; Brenda Polan, then at the *Guardian*, who responded to my plea for wider recognition of the needs of the young bereaved by printing my article on the subject; Derek Nuttall, former Director of Cruse, who gave much useful information; and Dr Gary Jackson of the Psychiatric Department at the Middlesex Hospital. Also thanks to Rabbi Jonathan Romain at Maidenhead Synagogue, the Right Reverend Geoffrey Rowell, Bishop in Europe, and Peter Wallis at the Oxford Quaker Centre for explaining the positions of their respective religions. I am also greatly indebted to Reverend David Barlow at the Cheltenham Ladies' College for his infectious enthusiasm and unflagging commitment to providing better support and recognition for the bereaved teenagers in his care. Caspar Williams kindly gave me permission to quote from his Masters dissertation on bereaved teenage boys. Julie Van-de-Vyver at the University of Kent provided much-appreciated assistance in researching this new edition. James Watson at Taylor & Francis has been a model of editorial patience throughout. Above all, thank you to all the individual men, women and children who have shared their personal experiences of losing a parent with me over the years, in person and by letter. Without them this book would not have been possible.

FOREWORD

Colin Murray Parkes

When it was first published, in 1992, Rebecca Abrams' book *When Parents Die* was blazing a new trail. Although much research into bereavement had been carried out, and much had been written, most of this output had focussed on the death of a spouse. Indeed, widows had become the model for grief. Abrams' work not only opened the door to understanding and helping people whose parents had died, it also stimulated research into a field that had been neglected.

Since that time a great deal has changed, much-needed research has been carried out, bereavement services have been improved, and an increasing number of parent-bereaved people have been helped; so much so that Britain's largest organization for bereaved people, *Cruse Bereavement Care*, which started as *Cruse Clubs for Widows,* now receives more requests for help from people who have lost a parent than it does from widows.

In successive editions of *When Parents Die,* Rebecca Abrams has kept up to date with this research while remaining true to her original assumption that the best lessons about bereavement are those given to us by bereaved people themselves. Abrams has been talking to and helping parent-bereaved people for over twenty years and her experience is unmatched. Indeed, she wears her knowledge lightly and makes no attempt to burden her readers with erudite details of research findings and theoretical models. Instead, she provides us with insights and solutions to the numerous problems and distressing feelings to which the death of a parent can give rise.

One of these problems is the general assumption that, because most of us will lose a parent sooner or later and few people are still dependent on their parents at that time, the bereaved will come though their grief without the need for the sympathy and support that is accorded to people suffering other forms of bereavement. Even the funeral gathering is an opportunity for friends and family to get together and may turn into a jolly party. Those most affected find themselves passing round the drinks and anyone who cries is an embarrassment. Bereaved children then feel guilty if they cried and equally guilty if they didn't.

And while it is true that most of us are better prepared for the timely death of an elderly parent than we are for untimely deaths, such as that suffered by the 18-year-old Rebecca Abrams when her father died, this does not mean that we can take it in our stride. Just as parents continue to think of us as children and treat us that way, so we all carry, somewhere within us, the secure confidence that Mum and Dad will always be there to look after us if the need arises. The death of parents, more than any other loss, moves us, abruptly, to the head of the queue.

At which point I am tempted to leave you in the capable hands of our author. But even Rebecca Abrams is no substitute for a parent for, as she reminds us: 'One of the hardest lessons that I had to learn was that no one in the world was more responsible for me than I was for myself. ... Once you can accept it, responsibility for yourself can bring with it a tremendous sense of relief and of freedom: you are in charge.'

Dr Colin Murray Parkes OBE MD FRCPsych is Emeritus Consultant Psychiatrist to St Christopher's Hospice, Sydenham, UK. He was formerly Senior Lecturer in Psychiatry, The Royal London Hospital Medical College, The Tavistock Institute of Human Relations, and Honorary Consultant Psychiatrist, St Joseph's Hospice, Hackney, UK. Dr Parkes was formerly Chairman, and is now Life President, of *Cruse Bereavement Care*, the UK's largest bereavement charity. He is the author of numerous publications on bereavement including *Love and Loss: the Roots of Grief and its Complications* (Routledge, 2006), and *Bereavement: Studies of Grief in Adult Life* (4th edition with Holly Prigerson, Routledge, 2010). In June 1996 he was awarded an OBE by Her Majesty The Queen for his services to bereaved people.

INTRODUCTION

This book is an account of my experience and the experiences of many other people who have had to come to terms with the death of a parent and the turmoil death has caused. The voices in this book are sometimes those of professionals, but far more often they are the voices of ordinary people whom I have chatted to, interviewed and professionally counselled over the last thirty years. My initial qualification for writing this book was personal experience. My father died when I was 18 and my stepfather when I was 20. Their deaths were the start of a lonely, difficult time which extended into every area of my life, affecting the way I felt about family, friends, home, school, university, work, and life in general. The experience revealed to me all too clearly how little support there was for people, particularly young people, struggling with a parent's death.

I wanted to write this book because when my father and stepfather died no such book existed, because there was nothing available that spoke to me about my particular loss or helped me to deal with my particular grief. Reading about widows, widowers and single parents helped a little, but not much: their situation was not my situation. I wanted to know if what I was going through was normal. I wanted to know that somewhere out there someone understood.

No matter what age you are, the death of a parent is always shocking. It is both a common experience, something that most people go through at least once in the course of their lifetime, and also an utterly unique experience. No one else will ever have had the relationship that existed between you and your parent, not even brothers and sisters in the same family. A parent's death is particularly unimaginable since we are given no prior experience of living without them. When someone has been part of your life for all of your life, it is virtually impossible to prepare for their death in advance. Even when you seldom or never see a parent, perhaps because of a divorce or a quarrel or geographical distance, there is still a qualitative difference between that kind of absence and the unending and irreversible absence of a parent who has died. Yet because the death of a parent is as inevitable as it is unimaginable, the highly personal meaning for you of *your* parent's death can easily be discounted by other people. The huge gap that has opened up in your life remains invisible to everyone else.

For young people, in particular, there are a range of very specific problems to face when a parent dies, problems which are still often ignored or unrecognized. A great deal of what children and young adults experience applies equally to older readers, but the particular problems facing people bereaved in childhood, adolescence and early adulthood still deserve more attention than they are currently getting.

In the UK a child is bereaved of a parent on average every thirty minutes. As many as 92 per cent of children in the UK will experience a significant bereavement before the age of 16.[1] In America, 1.2 million children lose a parent to death before age 15,[2] and 1.9 million have lost one or both parents before they are 18.[3] For young people, all the 'normal' difficulties of losing a parent are compounded. You are unlikely to have friends who've been through the experience themselves, and it is therefore often the case that the people you normally turn to for support won't be able to help or understand what you're going through. You may have had no previous experience of bereavement yourself, and be as baffled as your friends by what is happening. Family, far from being a source of support, can often be the cause of additional pressure, and seeing the people you love in pain can also be extremely hard to handle. On a purely practical level, the hectic timetable of youth leaves little space for grief and grieving: essays and exams don't wait because you are depressed and not sleeping; job interviews can't be put off because you are still in mourning; the new term starts whether or not you are ready to face it. Teachers, trained to teach, may have little idea how to help a bereaved pupil or what to say to him or her; not infrequently teachers and other adults make matters worse by adopting a 'business as usual' approach, happy to believe that the young are resilient and that time will heal. That may be true for some young people, but certainly is not true for all. It can, and often does, add to the acute sense of isolation and loneliness that young people feel after a parent has died.

Death is not in the scheme of things at this time in your life. It is usually premature and unexpected. It sets you apart from your friends, and places a burden of emotions, expectations and responsibilities on your shoulders that you are not at all ready for. Not being prepared for a death or its effect on your life makes it all the more shocking. It can leave you feeling that the whole world has become an unsafe and unreliable place in which nothing can be trusted or valued any longer.

A parent's death makes you different from everyone else of your age, and makes it difficult to do things that are normal for people of your age; in short, it interferes at every level with the business of being young and growing up.

A parent's death when you are in your teens and early twenties creates impossibly conflicting needs: you expect to be leaving home, moving out into the world, separating from your family, but a parent's death makes you less inclined to do those things, less confident, more fearful, more inward-looking. Should you leave home or stay home? Should you care for a remaining parent and siblings, or leave them, as planned, and get on with your own life? Should you take on new challenges or shun them? You can feel left behind, but unsure how to catch up. The great rush into adulthood rarely waits for those who are grieving for a parent.

Your perspective on life in general can be seriously affected by a parent's death, and your feelings about the many changes that are taking place at this stage in your life may be radically altered too. Saying good-bye to family, friends and familiar places can arouse painful feelings of loss; it can feel an unbearable wrench, not the exciting adventure and opportunity it should be – and still is for others. Friends seldom know how to help and their ignorance can make them insensitive and incompetent. This, combined with the misconceptions of older people, means that young people are often left with very little support, inside their families or outside them. Loneliness is a problem for anyone coping with bereavement; for young people it is particularly bad. Common feelings of isolation and abandonment are often made worse by lack of formal support and recognition. One small example: how many people think to write condolence letters to the children of the deceased?

Perhaps the hardest aspect of a parent's death for young people – and the one most consistently overlooked and misunderstood – is that death, mourning and grief involve feelings of helplessness and lack of control that are exceptionally difficult to cope with when you are at precisely the stage in your life when you need to feel confident and in control, at a time when everyone expects you to be taking charge of your life – yourself included. Immense pressures on people in their teens and early twenties often make it *impossible* to grieve. There simply is not enough time, energy or emotional strength to cope with everything. For young adults the struggle is not only how to cope with the bereavement itself, but also how to cope with it in the context of an unaccommodating world. Often the only solution, the only effective strategy for survival, is to put it off, get through the next day or week or month and deal with grieving later. Grief is delayed not because of inadequacies on the part of the individual, but rather because of a difficult combination of the developmental stage you are at and the often insensitive and unsupportive environment in which you are obliged to do your grieving. Delayed grief is very common for young people who have lost parents, yet grieving can no more be avoided than death itself. For young bereaved people, as a result, grief delayed can easily become grief denied. Not surprisingly, suppressed and delayed grief accounts for many of the problems experienced in adulthood by those bereaved in childhood and as teenagers.

Understanding at least a little about the process of mourning the death of a parent can help to buffer young people from some of the long-term problems associated with bereavement. It can help you to make sense of what you are going through, and help you to find a place for death in your life at an age when you are expected to be lively, optimistic, care-free; when you are expected to take risks, leave home, get jobs, be sociable, believe in the future, fall in and out of love; at an age when death makes all these 'normal' things seem very difficult, impossible even. It can help you to make sense of the experience of being bereaved when you are halfway between being a child and being an adult, when you are young and old, and when life was confusing enough already without the added complication of death.

Since *When Parents Die* was first published in 1992, I have received a great many letters – brave, inspiring, sometimes heartbreaking letters – from people of all ages, who have written to share their experiences of isolation, depression, confusion, guilt and rage following a parent's death. Some of these people had only recently been bereaved and were still in the early stages of mourning, others were writing about a death that had occurred many years before. Regardless of when their parent had died, they wrote so poignantly and vividly of their loss that no one reading those letters could be in any doubt about the profound and often cala-mitous impact of a parent's death. Again and again they told of lack of support and solitary anguish. So many people so overlooked for so many years. I was grateful that they had taken the trouble to write – their letters confirmed my conviction that there was a great and unmet need for support after a parent's death – and I was deeply moved by the stories they related: one woman, now in her forties, wrote of having had to sit an important school exam the same morning that her father died; a 19-year-old described the difficulties he was having with his first term at university only weeks after his mother's death. The recurring themes of the letters closely mirrored my own experience: the acute loneliness; the lack of understanding from other people, even close friends; the uninten-tional insensitivity of teachers and employers; the internal and external pressure to 'get over it'. These are also themes that I have encountered repeatedly in my work as a bereavement counsellor with Cruse and at the Cheltenham Ladies' College, and in countless conversations over the past three decades with people coping with the death of a parent or working with those who have lost parents.

What really surprised me about the letters, however, was the age range of the people writing them. While this book was intended primarily for readers in their teens and early twenties, it was actually being read by people of all ages, some of them well into their sixties and seventies. These letters were proof, if any were needed, that the death of a parent is not something that becomes easier with age, nor is it a loss that automatically fades with time: on the contrary, a parent's death stays with you and shapes you for the rest of your life; it becomes a part of who you are, like having blue eyes or black hair.

The second edition of *When Parents Die*, published in 1999, was in large part a response to the need so palpable in the many letters I received after the book's first publication. It expanded the scope of the original text to speak to children of all ages who'd lost a parent, whether they were 6, 16 or 46. It was also a reflection of how my own understanding of grief and loss had changed as I myself was changing. When I first sat down to write this book, I was in my late twenties, still single. When I wrote the second edition, I was in my mid-thirties, married with two children, a parent myself, acutely aware of what my death might mean to my children, aware too of how parental death had affected the kind of parent I was. I was increasingly conscious that grief was not a one-off event, but a life-long process; not one adjustment, but a series of adjustments made over the course of many years. The cycle of life does not end with death, but spins ever onwards. As it does so, it continually provides us with occasions to revisit our relationships with those who have died and with those who live on, with fresh perspectives and insights.

This third edition of *When Parents Die* draws on and benefits from two important developments that have occurred in the past decade: first, a major shift in the theoretical understanding of mourning; and second, a wealth of recent research into the specific impact of parental loss. Both of these underpin and inform this new edition in fundamental ways.

Since the appearance of the second edition, theoretical understanding of the grieving process has undergone a major sea change, driven in large part by the work of Phyllis Silverman and Steven Nickman at the University of Harvard on 'continuing bonds'.[4] Long-established theories that conceptualized grieving as a series of discrete stages leading within a fixed time frame to recovery from a loved one's death have been largely superceded by a far less time-bound view of grieving, which instead envisages the bereaved person as embarking on a highly individualized journey through a range of emotional tasks that lead gradually and often unpredictably to a state of acceptance of loss. The emphasis in current thinking about grief and grieving is on forging a continuing relationship with the person who has died, rather than on working towards an emotional amputation of that person from your life. Before I came across the 'continuing bonds' theory of grieving I was struggling to fit the round peg of my own experience of loss, and those of the people I was working with professionally, into the square peg of the theory. It wouldn't go. I knew something was wrong with the theory, but had only my own instinct and a small number of case studies to go on. Tentatively I suggested that 'letting go' was perhaps not the holy grail of grieving it was held up to be. Encountering the work of people such as Silverman and Nickman was a vindication of my instincts and a validation of my own observations. More importantly, their work was grounded in robust research conducted over many years. In the past decade their ideas have moved steadily into the mainstream of work with bereaved people. The impact has been little short of revolutionary, both for bereaved people themselves and for those supporting them: it has given us permission to say and feel what we know to be true about the long and frequently un-straightforward process of coming to terms with the death of a parent.

The second major change since the previous edition is that, in the past decade, a significant body of research has emerged on the specific impact of parental loss on children and adolescents, and its consequences over time. A range of factors, including catastrophic events such as 9/11, the devastation caused to families by AIDS, and a steady demographic shift in the developed world to having children later in life, have all contributed to a growing awareness of and interest in the experience and needs of bereaved young people. Not only is there now much more understanding than ten years ago about the impact of 'ordinary' parental loss, but there is also a far greater sensitivity to the needs of young people who lose parents in 'extraordinary' circumstances. Different approaches to helping the bereaved young have been pioneered, studied and evaluated. Important questions about how young people grieve, how parental loss differs from other kinds of loss, whether girls and boys grieve differently, how age affects grieving have now begun to be systematically investigated, and important answers have begun to emerge. Where I had almost no research to draw on to substantiate my findings and conclusions in the first edition of *When Parents Die*, in this third edition I have encountered the opposite challenge: how much of the abundance of recent research to include. While the key points in the first edition about losing a parent remain fundamentally unchanged, certain aspects of parental loss turn out to be even more significant than I originally proposed, in particular the role of the surviving parent and the prolonged nature of adolescent grieving. The significance of age and gender have also emerged as important factors in how people grieve and how they adjust to loss.

When Parents Die remains at heart what is has always been: a book for everyone and anyone who is feeling or has felt the impact of a parent's death, whether or not they were bereaved two weeks, two years or twenty years ago. This is a book about making space for the vast presence of death without letting it engulf you in the process. It is about finding ways of keeping your dead alive without having to live as if you were half-dead yourself. It is about living with death at a time when your dead should still have been living. A parent's death marks the end of a life, but not the end of your relationship with that person. This is not an easy or effortless understanding to reach, but it is a vital one, and ultimately it is this understanding that can enable you, with time, to replace the shock of death and the pain of loss with a renewed sense of connection to and pleasure in life.

1

MY STORY

All happy families are alike, but an unhappy family is unhappy after its own fashion.

Leo Tolstoy

The opening sentence of Tolstoy's novel *Anna Karenina* rings unquestionably true for anyone who has experienced the death of someone they love. Every bereaved family has its own particular circumstances that make its experience of death unique. All families are complicated and death throws a spotlight on the complexities. This was one of the things I learnt after my father died: death did not tidy up things, it did not suddenly make everyone behave like angels, it just made them behave even more like themselves than usual. Death did not solve problems, it simply highlighted them. Even if outwardly a family appears conventional enough, behind closed doors there is no such thing as a conventional family. Each family is made up of individuals and will itself be individual in one way or another.

It is this sense of uniqueness, of isolation, that can make you feel so totally unsupported after the death of a parent. Suddenly there is a vast gulf between you and the rest of the world.

Your experience of a parent's death will be unique to you, but there will also be aspects of your grief that you share with others in a similar situation. My story, too, is unlike anyone else's, and yet it contains many moments, thoughts and feelings that other people will also have experienced.

I was 18 years old and had just got my A level results. I had done reasonably well (no As, but no Es either) and decided I would stay on at school for an extra term to have a go at the entrance exam for Cambridge. One Thursday at the end of October with a fortnight to go until the exams I was told that Cambridge wanted me to go up the next day for a pre-exam interview. Any confidence I had had disappeared completely at that moment. But in fact the interview went all right and that evening I rang my parents to tell them about it. First I rang my father. He was throwing a party for Hallowe'en and said he couldn't talk for long. He sounded very cheerful, a little drunk and as if he was enjoying himself. In the background I could hear the other guests laughing and talking. It was clear he was busy. I then rang my mother in Bristol. (My parents had divorced when I was a child and both had since remarried.) Afterwards I went to meet my boyfriend. We went back to his college and spent the evening in the bar.

The following morning we were woken at nine o'clock by one of the college porters banging on the door. He said my boyfriend had to ring home. This was years before the invention of mobile phones, and I went back to sleep while he set off in search of a phone box. Ten minutes later he came back saying that he'd spoken to his younger brother and in fact I was the one who had to ring home.

'Oh, can't it wait? I'm sleeping.'

'No,' he said. 'It might be something important.'

'It won't be,' I said. 'It never is. You know what my family's like. It'll be something entirely *unimportant*.'

'But it *might* be, you never know. Come on, *please*.'

What I didn't know was that my boyfriend had already been told what had happened by his brother, but hadn't the heart to tell me himself.

Eventually he cajoled me out of bed, and we set off for the phone box. It was a beautiful autumn day: clear blue sky, a light frost on the grass and the leaves of the chestnut trees shining gold in the sunlight. I chattered away. Tim held my hand but did not speak. The phone box was occupied by a girl who was having a long conversation with her mother.

'Shall I tell her I have to make an urgent call?' I said, never very patient.

'Yes, do,' said Tim, never one to make a fuss. Still I didn't think anything was wrong.

I dialled the number and my stepsister answered.

'Hi, Lucy, I just got a message to ring.'

'Yes,' she said. 'Something terrible's happened. Your Dad's died.'

'Oh,' I said. 'Oh dear. What happened?'

I thought she said the *cat* had died. Lucy was very attached to the cat, I knew.

'He had a heart attack.'

'That's awful. You poor thing … '

2

'I've been up all night ringing people,' she said.

Then I remembered the cat was female.

'*Who's* died?' I said.

'Your Dad!'

Apparently I didn't even replace the receiver. I just let it drop and left it swinging. Tim had to put it back on the hook. I couldn't see or think. I was just crying and crying, unable to stop. Saying the only thing that was in my mind, over and over again, repeating to myself, 'It's not true. It's not happening. Not *my* Dad. It can't be true.'

I didn't know what to do or where to go. My mother and stepfather had left that morning for a holiday cottage in the Lake District with my little brother and sister. My oldest brother, Dominic, was living in Canterbury and not on the phone. My stepbrother, Christian, was with his girlfriend in York. Finally I remembered family friends who lived outside Cambridge and rang them. They said to stay put and they'd come and get us right away.

While we waited, we sat in a vegetarian restaurant and had the unhealthiest thing on sale: chocolate cake. I was still crying, amazed I had so many tears in me. I can't remember if I ate the cake or not. The friends came in their car and drove us back to their house, where for the next few hours they kept us stoked up with cups of tea and allowed me to say whatever came into my head. At about four o'clock my mother rang. She had just heard the news and was driving back to Bristol immediately. At eight o'clock that evening Tim and I caught a train to Bristol.

That night back home everyone gradually began to arrive from various parts of the country. All I remember is the endless cups of tea, a sea of faces and an excruciating, crushing tiredness in every fibre of my body.

The first moment when it really dawned on me that my father was dead came a couple of days later when my aunt took me with her to the florists to order flowers for the funeral. The woman behind the counter asked to whom the card should be made out and I heard my aunt reply, 'To the late Philip Abrams'.

Two days before the funeral we all took the train from Bristol to London and from there north to Durham, where my father lived. Arriving at the house that evening was a tremendous shock. I could not stop myself from expecting to see his face around every corner, to see his large bulky figure standing in the doorway, or hear his friendly tuneless whistling on the stairs. The house was so much his house, so much part of him, that it seemed impossible that he should not still be somewhere in it. Never had it felt so inhabited by him as that evening when for the first time in my life it was not. Every stroke of paint, every picture, every piece of furniture, even the *smell* of the house was Dad. The overwhelming impression of his being there was increased by the fact that my step-mother had left everything exactly as it had been. On the desk in his study there were two lists of things to do, one for that weekend, the other for the weeks leading up to Christmas. In the bedroom, the yellow jumper Dad had laid out to wear the next day was still draped over the chair. Everything spoke of his presence, but he himself was not there.

Instead there were these other people, so many of them it seemed, all talking and milling about, busy and aimless at the same time. All I wanted to do was to think about and feel for Dad; instead I was obliged to talk and be sociable, to be aware of the other people and their angry outbursts, tears, and unfunny jokes.

More than anything I loathed the sanctification of my father, a process that began to take place almost immediately he was dead. I knew him as bad-tempered, difficult, antisocial, allergic to physical exercise. And I knew him also as clever and sensitive and great fun and mischievous. All of these made up the father I loved. It was terrible to hear him being turned into some kind of saint. People said things that simply weren't true. It all became quite laughable at times. I listened in amazement as my father was transformed into the kindest, nicest, sweetest person that ever lived. I am sure at times my jaw must have dropped in outright astonishment. It didn't help me at all, this enshrining in saintly characteristics. It merely increased the sense of unreality, the feeling that nothing was real or sure or reliable any more. And it increased my sense of profound isolation: the sensation that I was utterly alone with my loss and grief. No one under-stood how I felt, because no one understood what I had lost. How could they understand when clearly their memory, their experience of my father, was quite different from my own?

The funeral took place the next morning in the village church. The weather was perfect: clear blue sky, frosty sunlight, golden trees, very like the day he died. As we followed the coffin through the church door, I felt more scared than anything else. My brother and aunt and stepmother had organized all the practicalities: arranged for the autopsy, coped with solicitors, settled bills, put announcements in the papers, booked the cre-matorium and the hearse, arranged the funeral. All I'd had to do was get through the interminable days. Now we had reached the church door and I was terrified.

The funeral itself was a slightly farcical affair. The coffin-bearers were colleagues of my father's and four men of less strength and more different heights you could not hope to find. Keeping the coffin on a dignified level was quite a challenge. At the little village church they misjudged the proportions of the door and dislodged the garland of freesias placed on

4

the coffin-lid by my stepmother. Although the congregation filled every corner of the church, most of them were confirmed atheists. As if to affirm the sense of the hollow hypocrisy of religious ceremony, the vicar, who had not known my father, mispronounced his name. 'Our dear departed brother,' he intoned, 'Philip Abrahams.' A slight rustle of embarrassment ran along the pews. My brother and I looked at each other, sharing the thought that, at any moment, Dad might sit up in his coffin with a long-suffering look on his face and tell the vicar, as he had had to tell so many other people in his lifetime, 'No H. A-B-R-A-M-S. No H.' For a second we were both torn between collapsing in a fit of giggles and bursting into tears.

My head was full of the strangest thoughts. I couldn't help thinking how small the coffin looked for such a big man, and wondering if they had squashed him into it. Soon after that, only moments after being so detached and clear-headed, I began to feel bewildered by it all: the people, the flowers, the situation. I started to shake violently and then could not control my tears any longer. My brother put his arm round my shoulders and held me tightly throughout the rest of the service. Beyond him there was my 78-year-old grandfather, looking small and sad. The day before he had said, 'If only it had been me.' I hated being stared at as we walked into the church behind the coffin; hated even more being stared at as we walked out. I felt all the watching eyes as a kind of assault, invading me when I was at my most vulnerable. More than anything I wanted to run and hide.

From the church we went to the crematorium. There was no ritual, no meaning, no time or care taken, just a clinical, utilitarian procedure, terrible piped music and the sickly smell of warm chrysanthemums. A button was pressed and a set of curtains swung down in front of the coffin. And that was it. We filed out of the building and stood for a moment on the gravelled drive, blinking in the sunshine, dazed by this brutally abrupt ending to a man's life. Then everyone went back to the house and the rest of the afternoon was spent eating, drinking and talking. Some people ate too much; some people drank too much; some people talked too much. I recall wandering through the tide of bodies, not knowing where to be in the midst of this quasi-celebration. Some faces I half recognized; some were familiar but made strange by the circumstances; many were unfamiliar to me – there seemed to be so many strangers that day. All these people, and the one person I wanted to be there, not.

In the days immediately before the funeral there had been an awful, dragging aimlessness; an endless stream of neighbours, friends and relatives; a meaningless sequence of meals which we dutifully ate without appetite, and which we eventually looked forward to eating because at least food introduced some sensation into the vast numbness that had settled so smotheringly over us all. There had been so many people and so much talk, everyone offering their memories and producing a kind of cacophony of opinions about who and what my father had been, taking away the person I knew and replacing him with someone else: a husband, colleague, son. I wanted to shut out their voices and their versions. By the minute my father was becoming less and less substantial, vanishing away, until I feared there would be nothing left but other people's voices.

In the days after the funeral, however, I could sometimes forget that Dad had died, and remember instead that I had to sit my exams in less than a fortnight, and that there was an essay on Chaucer to hand in that night. Thinking about my Chaucer essay made me feel guilty, but trying to forget about it made me feel guilty too. I was obsessed with the desire to go round the house and gather up all the things Dad had ever given me and all the things I had ever given him. I wanted to take them with me. I kept thinking: 'All those books, all those records, all those pictures, letters, photographs ... .' I was terrified the whole lot would be sold or burnt or thrown away. I was worried that my stepmother might forget that I needed things, might not understand that his possessions were a part of him and that I might need something of him, to remember him by, to keep him with me.

Two days after the funeral I was put on a train back to Bristol. My exams were looming and I had to get back to school. It had been odd being in my father's house in Durham, expecting him to be there still, but it was even odder being back in my mother's house in Bristol. Everything was so normal – that was the oddest thing of all. There we all were, having supper, going to school, going to work, watching TV – as if nothing had happened. The very normality was strange; made me feel that there was no normality anywhere any more.

For the first few weeks my mother frequently burst into tears, my stepsister was also very tearful, but I didn't cry at all, and their outbursts made me uncomfortable. I simply didn't feel anything. There was no emotion. I was quite cold and dead inside. There was no sadness or pain, nothing concrete like that.

It worried me. Perhaps I had not loved my father? But I couldn't make myself feel what I simply did not feel, so what was I to do? Looking back on those weeks I remember how dark and gloomy everything seemed: the other people were like the shadowy figures in a dream, the rooms I moved through were grey and dingy. I had switched off my mind and my emotions. I had shut myself away inside myself.

The only clear indication that I was unhappy – and it was not clear to me at the time – was that I felt sick a lot of the time with a kind of nervous anxiety in my stomach. I didn't like this queasiness, I didn't want to know about it, I certainly didn't want to connect it with my father's death. Instead I began to overeat. It was easier to feel sick from too much food rather than from emotions that I did not know what to do with. Food was easier to explain to myself and to deal with: it numbed and distracted me from thinking about Dad and death, it reduced the frightening feelings inside me to a straightforward self-inflicted discomfort caused by too much bread or pudding. Without really understanding what I was doing, I was trying to replace by food all the troubling emotions I was stuffed with. And for a while it worked, but it established a new problem: the habit of avoiding difficult emotions. In many ways this avoidance tactic complicated matters, making it harder to reach my real feelings, confusing the already confusing business of my father's death with other confusing matters of diet, calories, weight. Not knowing the trouble it would cause me in the future, seeking the short-term solution for now, I got used to ignoring my feelings and denying my needs. At a time when I badly needed to be loved and to love myself, I instead devised a way of hurting myself. As if I weren't full enough of hurt already, I had to pile on more.

At home, I was irritable and bad-tempered, especially with my stepfather, furious, I suppose, that he was alive at all. How dare he be alive and my Dad dead. I was rude and aggressive whenever the opportunity arose, and family mealtimes were soon unbearable with me picking fights and flying into a rage at the slightest provocation. Looking back, I can see how painful that must have been for my stepfather: he had looked after me since I was a little girl, undoubtedly loved me and wanted to help me, but the only part I would allow him was that of personal punchbag. Much of the rage I directed at my stepfather was, I later realized, fury with my father for having died and left me – and anger with myself for not having been able to prevent his death.

School was now difficult too. I had changed schools that term and had not yet made new close friends. When I came back to school after my father's funeral I felt lonely and awkward. The other pupils were awkward too, embarrassed to talk to me, not knowing what to say. I could see how much trouble they were going to, to avoid any mention of fathers or death, but the harder they tried to avoid these subjects, the more inevitably they would crop up. Once-innocent phrases like 'I nearly died' and 'I'm dead tired' and 'I'm dying to … ' had them blushing and squirming with embarrassment. Partly I felt sorry for them, but partly I was cross with them. Why should I have to deal with their feelings when they were being so hopeless in dealing with mine? Why should I have to make allowances for them, when they should have been making allowances for me?

The most baffling incident of all came on my first day back at school after the funeral in a lesson on the Romantic poets. The teacher asked me to read out a sonnet by Wordsworth called 'Surprised by Joy', a poem I did not know. I began to read aloud:

> Surprised by joy—impatient as the wind
> I turned to share the transport—Oh! with whom
> But thee, deep buried in the silent tomb ...

With a ghastly shock I realized what the poem was about. I read on:

> That thought's return
> Was the worst pang that sorrow ever bore,
> Save one, one only, when I stood forlorn,
> Knowing my heart's best treasure was no more;
> That neither present time, nor years unborn
> Could to my sight that heavenly face restore.

When I came to the end of the poem there was a silence in the room. I did not know where to look. Neither, it seemed, did anyone else. I did not know how many of them knew where I had been that week, what I had been doing. I did not know if the poem had shocked them too. I knew only too well, however, the feeling the poem described: that moment of wanting to tell someone something, to share an experience or thought with them, and then remembering that of course you can't because they are dead. I knew all about that shock of remembering what you had managed, amazingly, momentarily to forget. For a second I was entirely lost. Then the teacher said, 'Would you read it once more for us, please?'

Would I *what*? But what could I do? I started again, 'Surprised by joy—impatient as the wind ... ', but I was astounded by the teacher's insensitivity. What was he playing at? Had he forgotten? Had he thought it might add meaning to the lines, or enhance my reading of them? Had he intended it as a way of acknowledging what had happened to me? Or a way of forcing the others to recognize what had happened? I was too amazed to be really angry. I was almost amazed enough to think it was funny!

It took two months for the numbness that set in with my father's death to begin to wear off and for emotions to start to filter through. Three months after his death, in January, I was called back to Cambridge for another interview. It was strange to be there again: Cambridge was the city where I had been born and brought up, it was a city intimately associated for me with my father. That week I wrote in my diary:

> Being here is painful and upsetting. I pass a coffee shop where we used to have milkshakes, or a sweet shop where we always stopped to buy Liquorice Allsorts. Everything has memories and meaning. When the phone rings, I half expect it to be Dad – even in other people's houses. In the morning I hope there might be a letter in his big, loopy handwriting on the mat. I see a tall man with dark hair in the street and I half think it will be Dad.
>
> And yet all the time I never stop telling myself 'He is dead.' I never, never forget about him or about it. It's dreadful. I have so many regrets, so many causes to feel guilty. Above all I wish he'd known how much I loved him. Why did it never seem important for him to know that when he was alive?
>
> I feel depressed, pressured, hassled, surrounded by pettiness, squabbling, money problems and indecision about the future. And I feel depressed about Dad.
>
> It is as if I exist on two planes: on the surface I can think and talk about him quite calmly, and then I feel the other plane, beneath the surface one, slipping upwards. When a particular source of pressure is relieved, like after my exams or now after my interview, I can't stop the flood of despair at the thought of Dad's nothingness, my nothingness, in fact the nothingness of everything. Most of the time I seem to exist in a void of emotion, very superficial, extrovert, cold – and then suddenly I'm left stranded by a wave of feeling, shocked by how vulnerable and lonely I am.

If only someone had told me that it was normal still to feel wretched and confused several months after a parent's death. If only someone had taken time to explain that *telling* yourself a person is dead does not automatically put a stop to your hope and need that he or she is still alive. I thought I was going mad – to be so out of control of my own mind that when I knew he was dead, cremated, scattered, gone, I could still think I saw him in the street, or might receive a letter or phone call from him. The feeling of missing him, of having lost him – and a part of myself with him – were bad enough, but they were made much worse by my fear that I was going mad, cracking up under the strain. Why couldn't I cope? I asked myself angrily. Why was I so feeble and weak? Two months. I should be over it by now, shouldn't I?

In reality, I was in shock as well as in mourning, and many of my thoughts and feelings were symptoms of shock. If only someone had bothered to tell me that when it comes to grieving there are no shoulds or oughts, that it is different for everyone, that you are allowed to feel what you feel, when you want to feel it. We do not grieve by a rule book. If only someone had said to me, 'Two months is nothing. You'll be doing well if you stop feeling upset and confused after two years.'

Two years later, however, my stepfather died. When we first heard the news, my immediate thought was 'Oh God, not again! How can we stand to go through it all again?' But I soon learned that every bereavement is unique, the death of a parent can never be prepared for. My father's death in no way made my stepfather's easier to bear or understand, because the situation, the person and therefore the grief were all entirely different.

That weekend, everyone was away except my mother and me. My stepfather and little brother had gone up to Yorkshire to take part in a Fun Run to raise money for charity. My little sister was on a sailing holiday with a neighbour's children. My 20-year-old stepsister, Lucy, was at a David Bowie concert in London. Chris, my 22-year-old stepbrother, was staying with a friend, and my oldest brother, Dominic, was at his home in Canterbury.

We'd been having a lovely weekend, Mum and I, sitting in the garden, reading the newspapers, eating strawberries. It was one of those wonderful summer days when the air is busy with the quiet drone of aeroplanes and bees and distant lawnmowers. On the Sunday after lunch we settled down on the sofa in front of the afternoon film. It was a black-and-white classic called *Mrs Miniver* and our eyes were moist with tears from the first frame. As the hero's plane nosedived and it looked doubtful that he would return, we sat and snivelled and laughed at ourselves for being so soppy. Outside the sun blazed. The whole day was fused with a fat contentment.

Then the telephone rang.

I went to answer it and my aunt's voice said, 'Hello, love, can I speak to your mother please?' She sounded rather sombre and instead of going back to watch the film, I sat down on the stairs while my mother picked up the receiver.

There was a moment's silence while Maureen talked at the other end of the line, then my mother sat down heavily on the chair beside the phone.

'Oh God!' she gasped. 'No! What happened?'

All the warmth drained out of me and out of the day. It was as if a heavy cloud had abruptly blotted out the sun and light and warmth.

Suddenly it was icy cold and very dark in the hallway. I waited on the stairs, already wanting to cry, already very frightened.

Mum hung up and came – staggered really – to sit beside me on the stairs. 'Brian's died,' she said. Her head fell forward and she started to sob. We put our arms around each other and stayed there like that, clinging on to each other, for a long time. Maybe it wasn't for very long, I couldn't tell. All sense of ordinary time had gone, along with all sense of contentment. She cried. I couldn't. Somehow her crying stopped me. Eventually her sobbing subsided and she said in a flat, exhausted voice, 'I suppose we'd better tell everyone.'

Then we began the seemingly interminable business of telephoning all the relatives and friends who needed to be told. Saying over and over again, 'I have some bad news, I'm afraid, Brian's died.'

I couldn't tell if it seemed more or less real the more often I repeated those words. They came nowhere near to capturing the fact that he was dead, but somehow it was helpful and necessary to keep saying them, to keep telling people, to repeat again and again, 'He's dead.' It was a way of making it seem even a little bit real, as if by repetition we were drumming the fact into our own heads, in the same way we had once learnt our times tables.

When my little sister bounded into the hall later that evening, all excited from her sailing holiday, she walked into a room full of faces and knew at once that something was terribly wrong. She says she knew from the moment I opened the front door to her and was unusually kind and gentle. When Chris and his girlfriend strolled into her house that evening, the lodger called down from the upstairs landing, 'Someone's died. I think it might be your boyfriend's father', not realizing he was standing right there. Lucy was staying at a friend's flat in another part of town. No one knew the address and there was no phone. In the end we tracked her down by driving along several possible streets and asking anyone we saw if they knew her. There was something utterly terrible about destroying the contentment of each one of my brothers and sisters in turn like that. The whole thing was like a hideous dream. Except it wasn't a dream. The next morning, Monday, my mother caught the train to Huddersfield and returned in the evening with my little brother, Seth.

So there we all were, the summer shattered, sitting in the house, not quite knowing what to do. Not quite believing that all over again, for the second time in two years, we were gathered together because of a fatal heart attack. How could this be happening to us? It was almost too much to bear. We'd only just got used to the death of one father and now here we were grieving for the other. Just when we'd thought our lives were taking us out in different directions here we were, dragged

11

back to the very place and people we'd thought we were in the process of leaving.

And then there were the friends and neighbours who came and went ceaselessly, bringing food for meals none of us felt like eating, but which we all ate anyway, not knowing what else to do with ourselves. Often these people seemed far more at home than we. They sat and talked, chatting generally or talking about Brian. I wished they would all go. I hated the house being invaded by all these people with their trite comments and irritating advice. I hated the feeling that we were on display. It was all so undignified: to be a public exhibit at a time when we felt raw and exposed and vulnerable. But we had to be civil to everyone, smile and welcome them in, when what we really wanted to say was 'Oh God, can't you leave us alone?' Or at least, that was what I wanted. For my mother, I think, the attention and sympathy and chance to talk were a source of comfort of sorts.

I can still remember the dragging tiredness which made me long for sleep but wake unrefreshed; the oppressive heaviness that descended with each morning and which sat on my shoulders throughout the day, shifting its weight every now and then in case I forgot even for a moment that it was there. I recall mealtimes as particularly awesome, each one a gruelling routine that had to be performed. None of us had the heart to eat, even if we had had the appetite for food. Mealtimes gathered us all together and made us confront the grief in each other, made us look at one another over the plates and cups and knives and forks and see the pain in one another's faces. And at mealtimes particularly it was impossible to ignore the one person who was not there.

In my diary I wrote:

> The sense of general loss sometimes dims the sense of personal loss. I feel completely suspended, abject. All my personality has been wiped out by the incessant need to make meals, iron clothes. I am both mindlessly active and totally passive. I seem to be hanging, waiting, all the time, to be triggered into action by the sound of Mum crying, or the phone ringing, or the doorbell going. And to have to go through it all again so soon is awful. This time though it is worse somehow – there is no energy, no fight in me. Just a numb resignation which eats away. This time it is not my loss, it is the loss to us all which seems so cruel. I feel negated by it, wiped out, erased by the enormity of grief and pain.
>
> Since the funeral the house has felt oppressive. I feel dreadful every second I am in it, and guilty and anxious every second

I am out of it. And it all just goes on and on and on. There is no end to it. I see the fear in Mum's eyes. The sorrow in Ell's. The silent resignation in Chris's. It is just too much. It seems no comfort that we all love each other. I come face to face wherever I look with pain and sorrow.

When my father died in 1981, I was not really affected by other people's grief. I did not feel responsible for anyone but myself and I did not have to think about anyone but myself. My father and I had a difficult and unresolved relationship and his death left many tangled threads and loose ends which I had to find some way of disentangling and tying up, but it was basically just him and me to think about. When in July 1983 my stepfather died, the situation was entirely different. As well as my own feelings, this time I was very aware of how it was affecting Seth and Ellen, my younger siblings, then aged 9 and 11. Most of all, I was affected by my mother's suffering. I could not bear her sorrow, but because she turned to me for help, I had to bear it. She needed me, both to help her and to help with the younger children. When my father died, I wallowed in thinking about him and about me. When my stepfather died, I was almost too busy thinking and worrying about my family to think about how I was coping myself.

It has taken many years to understand my reactions to the deaths of my father and stepfather. I know now that some of the things I experienced after their deaths, and which made adjusting to life afterwards so much harder, could have been avoided had there been more help and information available at the time. Some of the difficulties I encountered were particular to me and my family, but many were common to bereaved children and young adults. Had I known more, had the people around me known more about the impact of a parent's death, the process of recovering and adjusting could have been made much easier.

Happily, much more *is* known now than was the case twenty or even ten years ago. Even so, I frequently meet people twice my age who are still struggling to come to terms with a parent's death, in large part because of the ignorance and unintentional harm caused by those around them. One woman in her sixties told me how her father had died when she was 15, how she had been considered too young to understand what was going on, kept away from the funeral, not allowed to come home until it was 'all over' – in short, given no room at all to express or resolve her grief. As she spoke the painful well of emotion was still there, forty-five years later, still able to bring fresh tears into her eyes. And it's not only young people who are knocked sideways when a parent dies. I recently met a man of 50 whose mother had died three years before; they had been very close and her death precipitated a profound life-crisis, from which he was only just emerging.

People are not computers that can be reprogrammed in a few minutes to accommodate new data. You cannot be expected to accept something so unacceptable as a parent's death within a few weeks, or easily and painlessly to adapt your life to such a massive change. It takes time to get used to an event that totally and irrevocably changes your life and perhaps your outlook on life. A parent's death is a common experience, something that happens to most people sooner or later. But it is also an utterly unique loss – no one else in the world has lost the same things that you have. Brothers and sisters may share some of your memories, but not all. How can they? Their relationship with the parent who died was, and is, different from yours.

The death of a parent can be a relief or a release for some people, but for the majority it is a stressful and distressing event in a person's life, especially when you are still a child or teenager.[1] Whatever age you are when your parent dies, remembering your parent is a vitally important way of understanding what has happened – to you and to them. When American researchers in Boston studied the way that bereaved children and teenagers thought about their dead parents, they found that those who allowed themselves to remember the parent who had died were more obviously upset four months after the bereavement, but far less distressed after two years than those who tried not to remember.[2]

Remembering is not always easy. For some, memories will be particularly painful. For others, remembering may be discouraged by those around them. But there is strong evidence that remembering is not something to be ashamed of or avoided. On the contrary: it is by remembering that we come to terms with what has happened. Each of us needs time to understand the uniqueness of what we have lost, time to make sense of it, and time to incorporate our lost parent into our hearts and minds in ways that allow us to engage positively and meaningfully in the day-to-day business of living.

2

FIRST DAYS, LAST RITES

I did not cry, because I still did not realize the magnitude of my loss.

Isabelle Allende

In the first few days after a parent's death, it is normal to feel numb and shocked. You may feel extremely tired, or full of nervous energy, unable to sit still or concentrate on anything for long. You may feel like being on your own, or you may feel scared to be alone. In these crazy days after a death, your whole world is in turmoil. The word 'limbo' means chaos, a state of being between two states, and this is exactly where you are at this moment: life without your parent has not yet officially begun (the funeral is part of this official transition), but neither is life with your parent officially over. It is a frightening time and a frightening place to be. Emotionally and physically, you are unanchored, drifting, not belonging, directionless, unsure of what is real and what is imagined. Everything happening right now seems unimaginable. You may also feel as if your life is suddenly filled with unwanted responsibilities, both for other people and for yourself. Older children, in particular, can find themselves having to make all kinds of decisions to do with the funeral arrangements, their dead parent's belongings, and a whole host of other practical arrangements. Having some idea of what decisions will need to be made and what the consequences of different choices will be, can help you in picking your way through the minefield of these early days. Take it easy on yourself; try not to rush into decisions that can wait for later; try not to take on more than you can manage, and try to take your own needs seriously as well as those of others.

In this chapter I will describe some of the ways of doing this by looking at the events that take place immediately after a parent's death and the dilemmas which you may face, such as whether or not to see the body; how to organize the funeral, and what to do about memorials for and mementoes of your parent.

Your experiences in these early days after a parent's death will vary a great deal depending on your age and position in the family. For very young children (under 5s), the predominant emotions will be confusion and anxiety.[1] The actual death may not make much sense, but the sudden disappearance of a parent is invariably the cause of very immediate anxiety and distress. A young child may search for the missing parent, ask repeatedly where they are and when they are coming back. The idea that a mother or father is never coming back is hard to understand at any age, but for young children the concept of death as finite and absolute is impossible to grasp. They will certainly be aware of the remaining parent's unhappiness and distracted behaviour, and will find it alarming and upsetting. Most young children will be openly upset themselves, crying and clinging, or else expressing their anxieties by being aggressive or naughty.[2] As well as plenty of love and affection, they need patience and kindness. They also need information. It is staggering how often adults omit to give small children clear, honest information about what is happening. One father told his young son his mother had gone on holiday when in fact she had been killed in an accident. The boy asked repeatedly when his mother was coming back and after six months of this, his father admitted that his mother was in fact dead. The boy became very distressed and, not surprisingly, his behaviour both at home and at school became disruptive and aggressive. That child's trust in the world had been deeply undermined, first by his mother's death and then by his father's well-intentioned but unhelpful dishonesty.

Slightly older children (6 to 9) will also feel very confused and anxious, but will be more aware of why they are feeling that way, more aware of what has happened and what it means. The younger end of this age group will still understand death in a concrete way. Physical evidence of their parent's absence, as well as physical reminders, are very helpful. Many adults baulk at taking young children to see and touch the body of a dead parent, but it can be the most helpful, direct way of helping the child understand what has happened. Similarly, it is nearly always helpful for children of all ages to attend the funeral, to see other people crying, to hear them talking about the person who has died.[3] It not only helps by giving them permission to express their feelings without shame or guilt, it also helps by validating their feeling that something momentously awful has happened. A great deal of research now confirms that hiding the evidence of a parent's death from bereaved children only makes them feel more alone with their sorrow and leaves them feeling deeply confused about what they are experiencing.[4]

As with younger children, clear and honest information is vitally important. A recent study of British adults who had lost a parent in childhood found that two-thirds had been told nothing at all or else had been given misleading or dishonest accounts of their parent's absence.[5] An 8-year-old girl whose adored father died of tuberculosis recalls, 'It was all hidden from me. I wasn't told.' Her mother could not bring herself to tell her daughter the truth, and eventually a neighbour told her, 'Your daddy's gone to heaven.' The little girl then asked, 'When will he be back?' and was told, 'Oh, you'll see him on Monday.' Now in her thirties, the legacy of this evasion is still distressing. 'Even now, to this day, I'm very bitter about my father dying. Very bitter. No one can answer you why, but I want to know why.'

How much children are told about a parent's death varies enormously from one culture to another. For many Europeans and Americans, the reason for not giving children information or involving them in the funeral is often driven by a fear of upsetting the child emotionally. In other cultures and ethnic groups, the reason may be more to do with beliefs about death itself. In many parts of Asia and Africa, for example, children are generally 'kept away' from the dead person and the funeral to protect them from 'death pollution' or spirits that might harm them physically. There is some evidence, however, that even where it is culturally normal to distance children from the reality of a parent's death, it can add significantly to their confusion and distress. In Zimbabwe, people avoid talking to children about death, and typically send them away to relatives until after the funeral. In a country where almost 1 million children have lost parents to AIDS, the stigma attached to the illness only makes matters worse. Far from helping bereaved children, the secrecy and evasiveness of adults creates additional problems.[6] One Zimbabwean girl whose mother and aunt had died of AIDS only found out later by reading the death certificate, against the instructions of her family. 'I hated everyone for a while,' she said, 'because they knew and didn't tell me.' Her 4-year-old cousin was also not told, and could not understand why his mother had suddenly abandoned him. 'He cries and keeps asking "Why is she gone?" He is very aggressive. He throws stones and pots for no reason.'[7]

Teenagers are more able to understand what death means – that it is irreversible and inevitable – but they also struggle with a devastating event that they are not yet emotionally prepared for. They often find themselves with no one to talk to about their parent and what they are going through emotionally, and in addition, struggle to cope with the rollercoaster of thoughts and feelings that are a normal part of losing a loved one. Teenagers suffer especially from feelings of loneliness and isolation after a parent's death. In adolescence, friends are immensely important, and the feeling of being different from friends, and unable to talk to them, is particularly distressing for teenagers.[8]

The insensitivity and lack of understanding about the feelings and needs of bereaved children means that important decisions in the early days after a death, such as whether or not a child should attend his or her parent's funeral, or how soon he or she should return to school, are still often made without any reference to what the child in question thinks about the matter. I have had letters from so many adults who found themselves in this position as children and are still trying to come to terms with their sense of exclusion years and years later. Even at the relatively advanced age of 18, I found myself with no practical role to play in the preparation for my father's funeral, because my older brothers took all that upon themselves. Their intentions were, I'm sure, completely kind, but have left me, nevertheless, with a sense of having been cheated, of somehow not having been included.

'Nobody asked me' is the feeling of many people who lost their parents when they were still children. It is a feeling that contributes to a general, and sometimes debilitating, sense of helplessness. Robert's mother died when he was 17. He told me:

> After mum's death, my dad and aunty took control of all the funeral arrangements, even the flowers from the children. I know they were only shielding us from the harshness of it, but I think it would have helped to have some input, even on a very practical level. Some suggestions I made to my dad about the service were ignored, and actually caused the funeral not to run as smoothly as it could have done.

Robert's instinct on this is correct: a major study of bereaved children in America found that attending the funeral and being involved in planning the funeral was one of the most significant factors in how well children of all ages adapted in the year after their parent's death.[9]

Older children in a family, on the other hand, can often find themselves shouldering a great deal of responsibility. You may find yourself needed and expected to share the burden on your remaining parent either by looking after younger siblings or by making decisions on your parent's behalf about the funeral arrangements. These extra responsibilities can be hard to handle at a time when you already have so much to cope with simply in coming to terms with the fact that your parent has died. The tension between your own personal needs and the needs of your family can cause complicated feelings of anger and guilt.

Conflicting emotions of this kind will very likely be present whatever age you are when your mother or father dies. Even children who are well into their own adulthood when their parent dies can find themselves treading through an emotional minefield, while also trying to cope with all the practicalities. The fact that there is no one to share the responsibility can be as unwelcome as having no responsibility to share. Work commitments, the needs of small children, the usual onslaught of housework – these things don't stop when your parent dies. The task of arranging a funeral, for example, would be quite arduous enough without the complexities of family dynamics that are invariably stirred up at this time.

Frances, a 60-year-old teacher in a state secondary school, was left in sole charge of arranging her mother's funeral after she died of cancer. Her younger sister was herself ill at the time and their only brother lived abroad. She felt intensely angry that all the arrangements should fall to her and her relationship with both her siblings deteriorated markedly. Her resentment stemmed in part from the fact that her mother's death coincided with a very busy time in the school year, but as a result of her siblings being unavailable to help, Frances was forced into a position of doing her job badly and letting her colleagues down. In addition, her only son had recently left home and she was finding his absence harder to cope with than she liked to admit. Her resentment also had a more personal source: a sense of unfairness, with roots way back in Frances's childhood, about the way she had always been cast in the role of the dependable daughter, which landed her with more than her share of responsibility, while her younger siblings pleased themselves. Frances found it very hard to focus on mourning for her mother with these powerful feelings of bitterness and anger coursing through her. 'John and Alison turned up for the funeral and I could barely bring myself to talk to them. Afterwards it was as if I had buried my mother without really noticing,' she says now, with evident regret.

How children of different ages conceptualize death and bereavement

How children and adolescents go through bereavement is linked to their cognitive developmental stage. The individual responses of each child vary greatly, but it can be helpful to have some idea of what it is appropriate to expect.[10]

2–7 years of age

Children at this age are naturally egocentric and believe that the world and other people feel and think the same way they do

Can't understand the permanence of death

Can't understand biological causes of death because abstract reasoning is not yet developed

However, a child knows about his/her own body and will try and feel what it is like to die. This can make them upset if they assume the death was painful

Children at this age are very vulnerable due to their limited cognitive ability

They may deny the death occurred or think the death is reversible

They may blame themselves and may think that their parent left as a punishment for something the child did

They will ask many questions about why and how the death happened

Socially children of this age will deal with death by isolation or acting out (hostile play) due to difficulty verbalising their feelings

May regress to immature behaviour: bed-wetting, thumb sucking etc.

7–11 years of age

Reasoning processes become more logical, but children of this age still struggle with complex, abstract situations

Child's egocentrism will cause a constant need to validate his or her own thoughts and feelings

Children at this age are able to comprehend the finality of death and how death may affect the child's own life

Children at this age may react to a parent's death by becoming socially and academically withdrawn

The child may internalize reactions to a bereavement at this age, e.g. by maintaining a relationship with the deceased in a fantasized world

They may externalize reactions, e.g. have angry outbursts, difficulty in sleeping, eating disorders, and persistent questions about the details of death

Due to egocentrism at this age, bereaved children are vulnerable to hypochondriac tendencies, shock, guilt.

Adolescents

At this age, children can understand death as finite and irreversible, but while comprehension of death is becoming more mature, mourning becomes more complicated by concurrent developmental tasks

Adolescents are psychologically striving for independence, while still emotionally and financially dependent on the family. Adolescents

are experiencing many physical changes, intellectually they are being pushed to do well to secure a good future. These normal developmental tasks of adolescence are often in conflict with the tasks of mourning
Conflict with family members is common after the death of a parent in adolescence.

Decisions, decisions

It seems very unfair that at a time when we are so shocked and unprepared for making important decisions we should be expected to make so many. The few days between the death and the funeral are crammed with tasks that need doing, plans that need making, choices that need taking. The additional pressure at a time that is already incredibly stressful can seem intolerable, although for some this activity may be a relief, providing a welcome distraction from the sorrow in the house, and an excuse to get out and do something.

James was 21 when his father died. He was pleased to have practical tasks to be getting on with, glad of the alternative to the sensation of helplessness. He welcomed the opportunity to escape the gloomy atmosphere at home, if only for an hour or two, and together with his younger brother took responsibility for arranging the post mortem (which must be done by law after an unexpected or sudden death); registering the death; putting announcements in the papers; cancelling credit cards and accounts; contacting solicitors; booking the funeral director; choosing the coffin. In short he and his brother busied themselves with all the paraphernalia that accompanies a death and a funeral.

For others, however, the endless demands may be an unwanted burden at a time when you want to be alone and quiet with your thoughts and feelings.

I remember hating the funeral director who came to our house after my stepfather died and sat in the front room asking what kind of tombstone we wanted. After him came the neighbours who all had questions of their own, and then there was the vicar, asking in his mild vicar's voice whether we wanted this hymn or that hymn. I didn't want any hymns at all; I didn't want a funeral; I didn't want my stepfather to be dead. I hated all these people for forcing us to make these decisions at a time when our minds and hearts were already so over-laden. Having older siblings I was not very involved in the practical tasks of arranging the funeral; my main responsibility was helping my mother decide what to wear and keeping younger siblings clothed, fed and occupied. I found this arduous enough: it was like being stuck in one of those dreams where you try to run and cannot, your limbs dragged down by some invisible and enormous force.

There is no right or wrong: what is important is to try to be as busy or as still as you personally need to be. If it is really impossible to meet your own needs because of pressure of circumstances or family demands, then try to be aware all the same of how you are feeling so that when opportunities do arise you can take them.

Seeing the body

One of the first decisions you may have to make is whether or not to see your parent's body. I had the option of going to see my father's body before the funeral. Frankly, the idea appalled me. The last thing I wanted to do was go and see a dead body – particularly the dead body of my Dad. Death frightened me. In fact, I only saw a dead body for the first time in my late twenties, when my husband-to-be's grandmother died at the age of 94. He was going to see her in the nursing home to say good-bye and wanted me to go with him. The situation was odd, to say the least, but it was not at all frightening. It has since become something of a standing joke in the family that Granny Spinney was 'not at her best' the day I met her.

Seeing my father's body was a different matter altogether, but I cannot say that I regret not seeing his body, because for me at that time it was the right decision to make.

Recently, however, a friend's father died and she rang me one evening to ask my advice: should she see her father's body or not? She half wanted to and was half afraid to. Would it help to see him dead, would it make his death seem more real? Or would she prefer to remember him as he was when he was still alive? Would she only ever be able to imagine him as dead after seeing him like that?

Although I turned down the chance to see my father's body, I have since talked and listened to many people about this, and my advice to my friend was to go and see her father. I told her what I have heard over and over again from other people – that it can be a relief to see the person you love. It can make the death seem more real. It can give you a few private moments in which to say goodbye, perhaps to say thank you or sorry for things done or not done. It can – many say – make you feel that the person you knew is no longer there. What you see is a body not a person. For those with religious faith or belief in the afterlife, this can be tremendously comforting: a physical sign that the soul has left the body and gone elsewhere.

The other side of the coin is that, yes, it can be very upsetting. To see someone once so vibrant and full of life now completely lacking vitality can be very shocking. Some people too do not like the change in appearance that can take place – a greyness to the skin or slight discolouration (perhaps even just the lifelessness of the body).

Obviously if your parent was killed in an accident of some kind or in other violent circumstances, or was wasted by illness, then the decision becomes more complicated still. Some find it comforting to recognize something of the person they knew and loved. Others will prefer to remember the person as they were in life.

For those people unfortunate enough to have to identify the body for legal reasons, there may be no comfort at all in the procedure. On the contrary, it may be harrowing, shocking, deeply disturbing. The only advice in this situation is to accept how frightened you may feel beforehand and how shocked you may feel afterwards. It is understandable that you should feel this way and it is not something to be ashamed of. Accepting your fear or distress will help to protect you a little from the additional burden of guilt and self-blame that might otherwise become a problem.

Where there *is* choice, it is important to realize that here again there is no right or wrong. It is an individual matter and ultimately at such times as these you should not do anything that makes you any more unhappy or uneasy than you already are. This is a time for doing everything within your power to help and care for yourself. Deciding whether seeing your dead parent will help or not is something that only you can do. It is irrelevant what anyone else thinks or does. You must do only what is right at this time for *you*. For my friend, seeing her father's body was the right thing to do. She rang afterwards to say it had been upsetting, but that it had also helped her. She was glad she had decided to go. For her it was the right decision. For you, it may not be.

Organizing the funeral

The funeral is usually the main focus of attention in the days after a parent has died and will generally take place within a week of the death, although the time lapse will vary. If, for example, key relatives have to come from abroad this may mean delaying the funeral for a while. The particularly difficult circumstances of the body being missing or unidentified will also cause delay. Your family's religion will make a difference: Jewish funerals are held between one and three days after the death with a short service, while a Catholic funeral might take place after seven days with a service lasting an hour or more.

23

In his excellent book, *Funerals and How to Improve Them,* Dr Tony Walter emphasizes how much choice is available when it comes to organizing a funeral: you do not have to have a religious service; you do not have to have hymns; you do not have to have a professional person to take the service; you do not have to have a religious building, a hearse or an undertaker. Legally, you do not even have to have a coffin or an official burial ground, although in practice other regulations make these last two pretty much unavoidable.

A funeral can be many things, but ideally, as Walter points out, a 'funeral must affirm both the universality and the uniqueness of death. We all die, but I die only once.' The funeral is not the be-all and end-all of mourning. A less-than-perfect funeral does not mean you will never again lead a normal life, just as a near-to-perfect funeral does not mean you will avoid any further sorrow and unhappiness. But the funeral is an important ceremony. It marks the passing of someone who has been precious to you, who has affected you, without whom you would not be as you are, and I would agree with Tony Walter that too many people put up with a ceremony that is unnecessarily unsatisfactory.

If you are in the position of having to make the funeral arrangements, some of the questions you might want to ask yourself are:

- How important is religion in your family? Is a religious ceremony appropriate for your other relatives, for the person who has died, and for yourself? If not, you might consider a Humanist service (see p. 214) as an alternative to a traditional religious service.
- Do you want to have the body prepared by a funeral director, or would members of the family like to do this?
- Do you want the coffin to be carried by undertakers, or are there relatives, friends and colleagues who would like to be pall-bearers?
- Do you want to have flowers at the service or to have money donated to a charity?
- If the funeral is going to be a large event, would you prefer to have a private funeral for close family only, followed by a separate memorial service at a later date for everyone else?
- Do you want the body to be cremated or buried? This will depend on religious belief; feelings about the existence or non-existence of an after-life; ideas about environmental responsibility. It will also depend on what you, the mourners, want to be left with after the funeral – a tombstone, a grave, or an unofficial site for the ashes which has meaning for you.
- Do you want a close friend or relative to talk at the service as well as, or instead of, the priest?

- Do you want the service to celebrate the life of the person who has died; comfort the mourners for what they have lost; emphasize the hope of an after-life or resurrection; stress the communality of grief or the inevitability of death? It can be all or none or some of these things.
- How best to involve the person who has died? By placing a possession of theirs on the coffin? By reading a favourite poem, or playing a loved piece of music? These small touches make all the difference between a personal and an impersonal funeral.
- Do you want a party afterwards? If so, do you want it at your home or at another less personal venue?
- How do you want to mark the place of burial? Do you want a tomb-stone or a plaque? Do you want the ashes buried or scattered? Do you want some kind of marker, such as a bench, tree or rose-bush?

Apart from these personal decisions, there are a range of legal and medical requirements. A useful guide to the procedure is published by the Consumers' Association, entitled *What to Do When Someone Dies* (see p. 233).

If you have the time and want to think in more depth about the purpose and type of funeral you want, Tony Walter's book cannot be recommended too highly. He talks at length about the role of the funeral, the pros and cons of burial versus cremation, ways of making funerals right, both for the person who has died and for the people who must continue living. He makes the point that the conventional crematorium leaves the mourners totally passive – as do most conventional church services – and that an advantage of burial is that there is at least some easy form of participation. Mourners can take an active role, either by carrying the coffin, or placing flowers or objects on the coffin, or simply by the traditional ritual of throwing earth into the grave.

These active ways of 'helping to bury your dead' make you feel less helpless, more in control, more involved. They affirm your links with the person who has died. They also help to establish that *you* are still alive, active, doing things.

The crematorium

Modern Western culture has invented the ultimate way of tidying up death: the crematorium. A loathing of the crematorium is the one thing that seems to unite everyone who has ever been to one, regardless of their closeness to the person who has died.

> 'Someone pushed a button and off he went!'
> 'Curtains came down in front of the coffin – like a Punch and
> Judy Show.'

'The crematorium was just one big chimney.'

'There was awful piped music playing. I couldn't believe it!'

'The coffin slid away on a conveyor belt. It was really dreadful.'

Unwelcoming, functional, antiseptic places, crematoria. I have seldom met anyone with a good word to say about them. But unfortunately, if the body is to be cremated, there are few ways of avoiding them. Tales abound of conveyor belts getting stuck or making horrible and all too audible grating noises as the coffin trundles away. One man told me how he found himself in a queue with two other groups of mourners, all of them allocated their five minutes. Last year I went to the funeral of an old woman, which was held entirely at the crematorium chapel. The grounds were not unattractive, with hills behind and green fields and trees on either side. The chapel itself was all right. But as we came out and were ushered round to the left, it was impossible to ignore the next 'party' filing in from the right.

Crematoria tend to be over-sanitized buildings, clinically tidy in procedure and place on the one hand, while on the other hand grossly insensitive to the feelings of the mourners and the significance to them of the person who has died. In trying to create places where nothing will offend, the designers of crematoria have come up with something that does nothing but offend. As Tony Walter puts it, '[A crematorium] burns bodies, but pretends not to: hypocrisy is built into the place.'

After his father's funeral – conducted mainly in a church but ending in a crematorium – Robert, who was then 23, broke down and wept. It was not good hearty sorrow, but a mixture of grief and horror at the bleak and perfunctory end to his father's physical existence. Robert was appalled that a man so precious and important to him should end in such a stark, ugly building devoid of beauty and meaning. My own memories are not much better. Above all I can remember the sickly smell of chrysanthemums – flowers I still cannot abide.

How to make the impersonal personal

Making the impersonal occasion of a typical funeral into a meaningful, personal event is often a daunting task, and one that in the midst of intense grief and shock you may simply not feel up to. This is particularly so if the family has not been religious but still decides on a religious ceremony. Events can quickly be taken out of your hands by other relations or professionals. An extreme example of this occurred recently when a vicar in Lancashire refused to allow one of his parishioners to use the word 'dad' on a tombstone, insisting instead that she put 'father'. While the vicar argued that the use of familiar and pet names was inappropriate on gravestones, which are public and historic monuments, he was over-looking the personal significance of a gravestone and its inscription to the bereaved individuals. Incidents like this can leave you feeling that the funeral had nothing whatsoever to do with your parent. The insincerity of the service in particular can sometimes be extremely painful, but there are ways round the problem.

When his father died, 30-year-old Dan knew that they could not have a religious service. His father had been a staunch atheist and was renowned for his strident views on the matter. Instead Dan contacted the Humanist Association who were happy to help arrange a funeral that was in keeping with his father's life and character, but which still gave Dan and his family an occasion to celebrate his life and say goodbye. 'Everything was right about it,' Dan recalled, eight months later, 'even the way the tape-recorder broke down – Dad could never in his whole life work a machine.'

It can be hard to make the service meaningful for you if your parent stipulated very precisely what he or she wanted. In these situations, the person who has died can sometimes be all too present, unforgettably and occasionally destructively so.

Marion was 21 when her father died. In his will he had specified that he wanted absolutely no ceremony whatsoever at his funeral: no mourners, no hymns, no prayers, no music, no speeches. Marion, her mother and her younger sister had no choice in the matter if they were to respect the dead man's wishes: he had stated explicitly that he did not want a personal funeral. Marion and her family found themselves in the peculiar position of having a funeral which was in keeping with the person who had died by being totally impersonal. 'In some ways it was entirely in keeping with my father's character, since he was a card-carrying atheist and rather eccentric,' Marion says, remembering the austere crematorium funeral.

> We went in, my mother, sister and me, no one else, and we sat there for five minutes and then we left. That was it! But I don't think it helped us very much; it made it difficult to focus on what we had lost. Recently I have been thinking that I would like to have a plaque or something. Very simple, but just something to let the world know that a special and unusual person lived and has died.

Marion's desire to have some sign that her father died is natural enough, and after ten years of feeling somehow denied the significance of her loss, owing to her father's strong opinions about funerals, she is finally acting on her need for some sort of marker, recognizing that her needs are more important now than his.

Marion's situation is unusual, but it shows how important it is to recognize your needs when it comes to the funeral. As Tony Walter puts it: 'A funeral says that something significant has happened, that a human life, *this* human life, has ended.' Even when circumstances permit, few of us will have the time, energy or inclination to start designing funerals; most of us have to make do with what is available. Nevertheless, there *are* various ways in which the fairly impersonal business of the conventional funeral can be made a significant event which will mark the passing of a significant person. It is possible to give most of the responsibility to the funeral director and the priest *without* relinquishing all hopes of individuality.

Suzanne is a journalist in her late twenties. Her father died of a heart attack one Sunday after they had spent the afternoon happily making marmalade together. His death came as a complete shock not only to Suzanne and her family but also to the community in which they lived. Her father had been an active member of the community and was popular and well known. Many people turned up for the funeral who were not related to the family but were connected to the dead man by some act of kindness or generosity on his part. The risk that the funeral might have become a rather impersonal event with many people not knowing each other was avoided by the priest's address. After speaking for a few moments about Suzanne's father, he then read out the obituary that she herself had written for the local paper. It was very personal, very direct and very moving. It brought everyone's attention back to awareness of the family's sorrow and loss. It focused everyone's minds once more on the man who had died.

Fifty-two-year-old Neil's mother's funeral was on an entirely different scale. It was a very small affair held in the chapel of the crematorium. Only ten people attended, reflecting the rather lonely person his mother had become. She had been a religious woman but not a churchgoer and the vicar was not known to the family at all. To make matters worse he bore an uncanny resemblance to Ken Dodd! The chapel itself was an ugly little building and when the sermon was over, a pair of curtains swished down in front of the coffin as if it were the end of a pantomime. The funeral however was entirely redeemed by the address which Neil had written for the vicar to read. Even the priest's buck teeth and flyaway hair could not distract from the passionate, honest and loving description of the woman now lying in the tiny coffin. It conjured up the image of someone of immense vigour, integrity, forcefulness, imagination and warmth. No one was unmoved by the celebration and the sorrow held in the words of the address. All present were for a moment able to forget the unfortunate surroundings and concentrate instead on a woman whose life was worthy of remembering and whose death was worthy of sadness.

Children too benefit enormously from being involved in making a parent's funeral personal and meaningful, as many studies now show. It is not only a case of making the funeral itself less alienating, it is also an important part of the process of adjusting to a parent's death in the months to come. Children of all ages can contribute to the funeral, through drawings or poems for their parent, which can be pinned up during the service, or placed on the coffin or in the grave. Some children will be comforted by the act of 'giving' a toy or other possession, or perhaps a photograph of themselves, to the parent who has died, so that they feel something of theirs is still with their parent and they are still connected in some way.

On the day

Even the most well-planned funeral will be upsetting on the actual day. As a priest remarked to me a few weeks ago, 'Funerals are much more complicated occasions than weddings, and we don't even get a chance to rehearse them!'

I remember how agonizing I found the drive to the church for my stepfather's funeral. The funeral car drove down the High Street so slowly, crawling past all the shops and the midday shoppers in their bright summery clothes. Inside the car we did not know quite what to say to one another; my brother cracked a joke, I think, and we all laughed. I felt painfully self-conscious, aware of the people on the pavement staring in at us, but aware too how irrelevant our grief was to them as they cheerfully set off as normal to buy apples and bread and shampoo. Usually we too were walking down the street at this time of day, off to the newsagent or the post office. Inside the funeral car we were so close to the everyday, literally a few feet away from it, but also immeasurably distant, locked up inside this big, black car with our knees squashed against each other's. The mixture of the mundane and the bizarre was confusing: the funeral car and the hearse in the midst of the lunchtime traffic and the people in their summer clothes.

Clare's mother had a Catholic funeral in Yorkshire in late November. For Clare the most difficult part of the day was after the service when the coffin was being lowered into the ground. It was a freezing cold day with a biting wind, and the graveyard had been turned to mud by the ceaseless, pouring rain. The women had to shift their weight constantly to stop their heels sinking into the ground. Everyone's umbrellas were blown inside out and no one was spared the cold and the wet. Their physical discomfort combined with the desolate, grey graveyard and the sight of her mother's coffin being lowered into the grave was hard for Clare at the time. Later, however, she felt that the austerity of the day was rather fitting: the elements matched her grief very well, 'as if they were angry and full of pain too', she says.

For some the hardest part of the day will be processing down the aisle with your family knowing that all eyes are on you. This feeling that your grief is exposed to the public gaze can be terribly painful. For some the shock of seeing the coffin will be the worst part. Others find they can be on automatic pilot throughout the service; it is only afterwards when they are surrounded by people at the customary funeral meal that they begin to feel unable to cope. 'I just couldn't stand it,' one 17-year-old said, 'I wanted to be alone and instead we had to have a party! I wished they'd all go home.'

Patricia was 42 when her mother died, after a short illness. Her father was already dead, and she and her sister were responsible for organizing the funeral, as well as all the other legal and practical business surrounding a death. Patricia, however, was so dreading the day of the funeral that she found herself unconsciously denying that it was going to happen. Her younger sister, Susan, recalls how Patricia refused to arrange funeral cars to take them and other relatives to the crematorium, saying they could drive themselves from their mother's home. She also insisted that they wouldn't need to provide any food for after the funeral, as 'there wouldn't be many people there'. Susan eventually asked Patricia's 15-year-old son to help persuade her sister that they would not feel up to the two-hour drive to the crematorium on the day, and that in all likelihood there would be over a hundred people at the funeral, many of whom would come back to the house afterwards, expecting both food and drink. 'Patricia just didn't want to think about it,' Susan says. 'I think she hadn't faced up to the fact that mum was going to die, and when she did die, she just couldn't bear it. But after everyone had gone and we were on our own, she kept saying what a good thing it was that we'd hired cars and caterers. She seemed to have forgotten that she hadn't wanted to.'

Displays of sadness and grief before and during the funeral vary enormously from family to family and from culture to culture. In some traditional Muslim communities, for example, it is expected that women will express their grief through loud crying and wailing, but not men.[11] In Balinese culture, strong control of emotion is respected, and displays of emotional distress are seen as dangerous and frowned on.[12] Children will tend to take their cue from the adults around them and the particular culture they come from. The Harvard Child Bereavement Study looked at the experiences of 125 children aged 6 to 17 and found that around the time of the death and the funeral, 42 per cent of children felt pressure to behave a certain way for the surviving parent's sake. Some felt they had to be restrained and not create problems. Others, particularly teenagers, felt under pressure to express their feelings more openly, and some felt disapproval from others for not crying.[13]

Whether open crying is seen as 'normal' or is disapproved of, the day of the funeral is invariably painful, and it is *supposed* to be: it is the first moment since your parent's death when you can focus fully on the fact that he or she is dead. One of the most crucial functions of the funeral is precisely this: to allow you to feel your loss and your pain. The formal emphasis of the occasion may be committing your parent to God's care; it may be to comfort the bereaved; it may be to make some sense of death itself, but the *private* function of the funeral is to let you concentrate for a while on the person you have lost and in so doing help you to start the process of finding ways of living with that loss.

Possessions

There is often a strong sense after a parent's death that your life is no longer based on firm foundations, that once-familiar people and places have become strange to you, and it is often accentuated by the loss of actual *things*. When so much in your life is in flux it is not at all uncommon to attach enormous importance to personal possessions. A brooch or a book or a photograph can give you at least something tangible that remains unchanged, something that makes you feel connected still to your parent. The business of disposing of a dead parent's belongings can therefore be extremely fraught and upsetting. Where there isn't a will, the division of possessions and property can be a lengthy process, which may add considerably to the distress it causes you and your family.

Depending on your age the ultimate say over what happens to possessions will usually be in the hands of your remaining parent or lawyers. This can exacerbate the feeling of being powerless, the feeling that your relationship with the parent who has died will not be valued by others.

Immediately after my father's death I was obsessed with the need to have things of his to remind me of him, to keep him alive in some way. I wanted to build a fortress of his books and clothes and pictures, and hide inside it. I needed my dad's belongings to make me feel he was still there with me. I was panicky with the fear that he would just slip away, vanish totally, that there would be no trace of him left behind. I was anxious lest my stepmother failed to realize how important my father's

31

belongings were to me, anxious lest other brothers and sisters took things I felt I needed.

It is not at all unusual after a death for people to react very strongly to the question of the dead person's belongings. Sometimes people are very reluctant to move anything at all. Occasionally this reluctance gets out of hand and people create a sort of shrine to the dead person's memory, at which they then worship. Sometimes the opposite happens: a widowed husband or wife will want to destroy, burn or throw out all evidence of the dead person, as if the pain occasioned by the presence of these belongings is simply too much to bear. If you do not feel the same way, this apparent desire to erase all trace of your dead mother or father's existence can be very painful.

Alan Silberberg, a Canadian writer, lost his mother to brain cancer when he was 9 years old. After her death, the family moved house several times and his father packed away his mother's belongings, and when he remarried, Alan's mother's possessions were given away to charity shops. As an adult looking back on his father's behaviour, Alan can understand his father's need to avoid reminders of his dead wife, whom he'd adored, and then out of respect for his new wife, his decision to get rid of those reminders. But for Alan as a child it was bewildering and distressing to have all trace of his mother's presence so rapidly removed from his life. In his wonderful children's book, *Milo and the Restart Button*, he writes about this experience and how hard it made it for him to mourn for his mother. In the book, Milo's father does the same as Alan's father, but Milo eventually decides that even if he can't have things that actually belonged to his mother, he can buy things from yard sales that remind him of her – a bottle of red nail polish, a kitchen timer shaped like an egg, a pair of sunglasses with big plastic frames. For Milo gathering together these objects is a turning point that allows him to remember and feel connected with his mother even though she is dead. As Alan Silberberg says: 'I had the character of Milo do what I wasn't able to do myself. I allowed myself to remember my mum. It was very cathartic, very healing.'[14]

Studies of bereaved children have also found that having possessions that belonged to the parent who died is an extremely important and helpful part of mourning, whatever your age. Over three-quarters of the children in the Child Bereavement Study had something belonging to their parent that they kept close to them – a tape of music they used to listen to together, an item of clothing, a baseball cap.[15]

While you may have to accept your remaining parent's need to do things in a particular way, at the same time it is important to recognize your own needs. You may not be able to prevent your parent getting rid of belongings before you would want, but don't be afraid to ask for something that you can keep, or if all else fails, you can, like Milo, put together a collection of things that remind you of your parent.

If you are in the position of being responsible for getting rid of your dead parent's belongings, think carefully about how you want to do this: should a collection of books be kept intact and given to a local library? Would a set of records make a good present to a school or hospital? Clothes can be thrown away or they can be given to charity. But try to hold off doing things in a rush. You may feel pressure to get everything back to normal as quickly as possible, but in reality you will find that it is a long time before that happens and the speed with which you dispose of possessions is not the determining factor. Most people find the time announces itself when it is right to do this painful kind of clearing out. Don't feel you must hurry up and decide. Out of sight is not out of mind, and the presence of possessions will not stop you and your family from feeling miserable, nor will possessions disposed of magically make you all feel better. In reality, holding on to a few possessions that remind you of your parent is likely to help not hinder your adjustment to their death.

If you possibly can, give yourself enough time in disposing of your parent's belongings to be ready to do so. When the time does come, it can be useful to get a friend to help, as the presence of someone who is not emotionally bound up with these belongings and their significance can help you to think more calmly and clearly about what to do with them, what you want to let go of and what you want to keep.

Memorials and mementoes

When the funeral cannot – for whatever reason – meet all the needs of the people involved, a memorial of some kind may provide another opportunity to do so. Objects that belonged to your parent are important for this reason too. Having something meaningful that belonged to your parent can provide you with a kind of small, personal memorial.

My stepfather was a great lover of English literature. He had been the only member of his family to go to university and with his first grant cheque had bought himself a proper big dictionary. This love of literature was something he and I had shared, and it was he who taught me how to read and understand fiction and poetry. He helped me prepare for the Cambridge entrance exams and was delighted when I got a place to read English. My stepfather died at the end of my first year at university; after the funeral my mother took me aside and quietly presented me with the dictionary. It is a very personal reminder of him and of my special connection with him through our shared love of books, and it is something I treasure very deeply.

Clothes, books, ornaments, a chair, a collection of old records, a photograph or painting – all sorts of things can be precious to you while meaningless to other people. My younger sister has a locket that she wore for many years with a photograph of her father inside. A friend has a skirt of her mother's; another has his Dad's football scarf. If there is something that you think could particularly help you to feel the person you loved is not irrevocably lost to you, something that you can have and cherish because it was his or hers, then I would urge you to ask for it. Private memorials are important to all of us, not a sign of morbidity to be ashamed of.

Sometimes you may want a more public form of memorial. This may be because a memorial service is expected, or necessary, in order to accommodate people who could not attend the funeral. It may be a way of having 'another go' at the funeral when there is more time to plan the event. It may be for entirely private reasons, or it may be a combination of all of these.

Joely wanted to organize a memorial service for her father. This was partly because the funeral had seemed to her inappropriate in many ways, not capturing her father's personality or achievements. The main reason, however, was that Joely's parents were divorced and her father's family had refused to let her mother attend the funeral. Joely felt very strongly that her mother should be allowed to mourn publicly the loss of her first husband, and that *she* should be allowed to mourn publicly with her mother. Organizing the service was difficult and upsetting in many ways, but despite the problems it did take place a year after her father's death and this time Joely's mother was there beside her.

Not having her mother at the funeral had somehow denied not only her involvement and connection with her father, it also somehow denied part of herself; at a time when one part of her was so lost through her father's death, it seemed vital to have the parts of herself that resided in still-living people, such as her mother, affirmed. As a public event it was not especially successful, but as a private one the memorial service was not only an opportunity for Joely to remember her father in a way that made sense, it also helped her face up to his death.

When my grandmother died, she left specific instructions about her funeral. She wanted an orthodox Jewish service at the crematorium where her husband had been buried. This was not entirely in line with her religious beliefs but was necessary if she was to be buried next to her husband, which was extremely important to her. My mother and aunt, however, agreed that *only* to mark their mother's death in this very restrained and somewhat impersonal way would not feel appropriate or sufficient. Three months later they held an event, a kind of party, to commemorate their mother's life. Numerous people who hadn't been able to make the funeral were invited. Various friends and family talked about the woman they'd known and loved. My sister played her viola, a close friend read a poem, another friend played the piano. It was a wonderful, uplifting occasion, in which a life was celebrated, rather than a death mourned. My grandmother's wishes had been respected, but the needs of the living had also found expression.

Public memorials need not be services: memorials can take the shape of benches, trees, plaques or even specific actions, such as the lighting of a candle. A memorial of some kind can be particularly useful if your parent was cremated or if their body was never found and there is no obvious sign to tell you where they are any more. Memorials are not indulgent, they are important ways of marking the significance of the person who has died, either publicly or privately.

Sara's mother was cremated when she died. The ashes were scattered in a graveyard and a rosebush was planted near the spot. Neither the rosebush nor the churchyard have any meaning for Sara and she sometimes regrets that there is no physical place where she knows her mother is. 'The odd thing is that it seems to matter more with time,' she says. 'As the awareness of Mum becomes less pressing inside me, I seem increasingly to want a firm sense of her being somewhere outside.'

Ann's father was also cremated. Her mother and older brother scattered the ashes from a mountain top in Wales, making the pilgrimage together in the memory of many walks and climbs they had made when her father was alive. Climbing this hill had been an achievement they particularly relished. Ann, however, had been too young to take part in these expeditions and therefore did not take part in scattering the ashes either. She could easily have felt excluded and been left with no clear idea of where her father now was, but after some discussion the family agreed that there was a need for a clear physical marker, and they decided to plant a tree in the botanical gardens of the town where they lived. Six months after her father's death, on a bitterly cold February day, Ann went with her mother and brother to plant a cherry tree in the gardens. Icy rain poured down and the gardens looked bleak and bare; the frail little stripling that the gardener planted seemed to capture all too well their own mood of frailty. But the idea of the blossom that would flower, and the leaves that would spring from the fragile branches, and the sturdy tree that it would, in time, become, was a comforting and inspiring symbol.

Trees are a wonderfully explicit symbol of the continuation of life, the process of growth and decay and regrowth, but they can of course be rather expensive. On the plus side, the cost of the tree includes the cost of tending it, which is probably comparable to the cost of upkeeping a grave or tombstone. Wardens of parks and gardens will usually be glad to oblige in helping choose a tree and a site for it, and they can also advise you as to the cost.

Benches are also a durable memorial, not indefinitely so – it depends on the type of wood used for the bench and the type of metal used for the plaque – but they are a good solid physical reminder of a person. Something about sitting on a memorial bench to a person you loved can make you feel very close to them physically.

Memorials can help ease the anxiety that if you are not careful you might accidentally begin to forget the person who has died, that they might just slip out of your existence now they are no longer alive. This is a problem many people share – how to keep the memory of the dead alive without having to keep all the pain of grief and loss alive too. A place where you know your parent 'is' and where you know you can go if need be, is a simple and effective way of doing that. Whether you decide to create some kind of memorial soon after your parent dies, or years later, memorials and mementoes are an enormously helpful and healthy way to keep memories alive while allowing sorrow slowly to subside.

3

DIFFERENT DEATHS, DIFFERENT GRIEFS

Death and the sun cannot be looked at too steadily.

La Rochefoucauld

Death is always shocking, no matter how expected it is, nor how long it has been coming. It is impossible to live with the full awareness of death's nearness. Even when a parent's death is inevitable, it is still not possible to be fully prepared for it. In order to cope with the probability of a parent's death in the near future and yet still carry on living, we *have* to dull our minds and emotions to death. It would simply be too painful to bear otherwise. Even if we know with a part of our minds, we stop ourselves from knowing with many other parts. It has to be like that, it is not a form of weakness or stupidity or false optimism, it is a form of survival. It is impossible to prepare fully for a parent's death, and however a parent dies it will always be a shock. In addition, the way in which your parent dies may affect the way you react to the death and also the way you are likely to mourn your loss.

This chapter goes through the different ways a parent may have died, including death after a period of illness, sudden death, and the particularly difficult event of a death by suicide. Sometimes a parent may have 'died' for you but continued living, for example after a stroke or through chronic alcoholism, or perhaps through divorce or separation. Each different kind of death comes with its own particular circumstances which in turn can affect the way you grieve. It can help to have some idea of what is 'normal' in your circumstances.

Death after a long illness

When a parent dies after having been ill for some time, maybe months or years, there is more time to prepare: you can talk with your parent about how life will be after their death, and how life has been before. You can do many practical tasks and to a certain extent sort out unfinished 'emotional business' with your parent. Organizations such as Winston's Wish in England and the Hospice Movement can and do help children and their families to cope with a long illness and to prepare for a parent's death. Winston's Wish runs courses, provides one-to-one support and also publishes a number of excellent booklets explaining the impact on children of a parent's death after a long-term illness.[1] Giving children age-appropriate information and giving them space to express their feelings clearly can make the anguish of slowly losing a loved parent somewhat easier to bear. But in practice, the 'preparation time' that a long illness *appears* to provide is not always easy to use in such a positive textbook way. It is *never* possible to prepare entirely; death cannot be totally prepared for in advance.

Jenny discovered this when her mother died of cancer. A malignant lump on one of her mother's breasts had been diagnosed when Jenny was 15 and the whole breast had had to be removed. After her mother's first operation, life at home changed drastically and never got back to normal. Weakened by the operation and depressed by the loss of a breast, Jenny's mother became irritable, anxious and easily tired, not the calm pillar of strength she had previously been. The treatment also made her feel very ill and exhausted. Over Jenny and all her family hovered the constant, unspoken and unspeakable fear that the cancer might have spread. A year later, despite all their hopes that the cancer had been caught in time, investigations showed the cancer had returned and was now in the spine, liver and kidneys.

Those months, between the probability that her mother would die and the day in May when she finally did, were something close to hell for the whole family. Apart from the invisible threat of the cancer itself, there were the side effects of the chemotherapy to cope with. Jenny found the physical change in her mother extremely distressing. Listening to her mother throwing up after every meal; watching her lose her hair, lose the colour in her cheeks, lose the sparkle in her eyes, lose so much weight that eventually she was unable to sit or stand without help, unable to sleep at night, and totally dependent on painkillers; watching her home fill up with ugly, frightening medical equipment, pill bottles and syringes; watching the slow, excruciating process of a life being destroyed, of a dearly loved parent being inexorably ravaged from within – these things were devastating.

How *could* Jenny get on with her daily life and see these things? It would have been like staring into the headlamps of an oncoming car. To survive herself she had no choice but to step out of the way and only glance at the headlamps occasionally. She adjusted to all the upheavals and changes to her home life, accepted the added responsibilities that fell to her because of her mother's illness. She even made herself talk about the 'cancer'. But it was still terrifying – the prospect of life without her mother. Already Jenny's mother was no longer able to do so many of the things she always had, from ironing their clothes; making meals; persuading them to do their homework or wash their hair; reminding them to clean the bath; looking after them when they were ill; offering her opinion on clothes, boyfriends, bedtimes. Jenny missed her already, but she shut out thoughts of how much more she would miss her in the future. Her mother was going to die; in her worst moments Jenny realized this, but she wasn't dead yet. As long as her mother was alive, Jenny held on to the small and dwindling hope that she might recover. Every remission revived that hope. Every relapse destroyed it. Life for Jenny in these two years was like suddenly being strapped onto a rollercoaster and trying vainly to carry on as normal.

In some circumstances there can be advantages to a death coming after an illness, because at least you may have had time to 'rehearse' what will happen in the future, either by discussing it with your family or simply by imagining how it will feel to come home from school, or go on holidays, or hear important exam results, or get married *without* the parent you love being there. This kind of rehearsing is often extremely upsetting, but it can also be very helpful. The hospice movement has raised awareness of how useful this rehearsing can be, and hospices play a very important role in helping people who are dying and their families to discuss and come to terms with not only the death of a loved one, but also what will happen afterwards.

When 10-year-old twins, Louise and Anthony, were told that their mother was going to die of cancer, they were closely involved in very practical discussions about what would happen to them in the future. Since there was no family member with whom they could live, they took the unusual step of advertising in the paper for a 'new' mother. In the months leading up to their mother's death, they got to know the family that would be adopting them, meeting on numerous occasions with their future adoptive mother and their own mother. They were able to raise some of the many questions in their minds and, most importantly of all, they were able to take a key role in determining what would happen to them after their mother died. Neither the fact of her tragically early death, nor witnessing the illness she had to endure, were any the less painful for her children because of these preparations, but at least Louise and Anthony were enabled to consider their future and to play a definite part in it. Instead of having to endure a drastic disruption from their past life, as so many children do, Louise and Anthony were given a crucial chance to build the beginnings of a bridge between their past and their future.

Louise and Anthony's story is unusual in many respects. Younger children generally are not given sufficient information about a dying parent's illness, or involved in discussions about what will happen afterwards. Because of their age, it can be very difficult for them to understand that their parent is dying, and more difficult still to handle the feelings this causes. Preparing for a future without their parent is almost impossible. In *Milo and the Restart Button*, Alan Silberberg writes about Milo's experience of his mother's illness and how it isn't until he goes to see her for the last time in hospital that he really begins to face what is happening:

> We walked into the room and I saw her surrounded by the pea-patch blanket. And she didn't see us yet and she wasn't smiling. She looked so sick, and as soon as she realized we were there, she tried to smile but I could tell she was faking it for us. ... That's when I found out she was going to have an operation to fix everything in her brain. And I guess we were there to wish her luck – but I felt stuck and frozen and didn't know what to do. If I knew that would be the last time I had to say anything to my mom, I would've said more. I would've said 'I miss you.' I would've said, 'I love you.' I would've said, 'Please come home and make me supper and I don't care even if it's fish – I'll eat it and never complain again.' I would've climbed into that hospital bed with her and pulled the pea-patch blanket over both our heads and hugged her so tight ... But I couldn't do any of that. I just stood there silent and stared at the blanket that would always be hers.[2]

Whatever your age, it is very hard to live with a dying parent. If you are old enough to understand what is happening, it is impossible to ignore not only the mortality of your parent, but also the acute awareness that you too are mortal and will one day die. To deal with this increased awareness of mortality, you may have had to 'shut down' inside. You may well have experienced many of the emotions associated with bereavement *before* your parent died: anxiety, denial of their death, anger, fear. If the illness lasted a very long time, or if you have found these emotions particularly hard to tolerate, you may have withdrawn emotionally as a way of coping with the situation – and this is often the case for younger children too. Emotional withdrawal can be helpful up to a point, but it can mean that once the person does die, you can be left feeling very locked up inside yourself, unable to feel anything, terrified of feeling anything because there is now so much to feel, like a great tidal wave of emotion pressed up against the dam gates. If this is so, you may need the help of a therapist or counsellor to find ways of letting your feelings out in a safe, manageable way.

Hope Edelman was 17 when her mother died. In her book, *Motherless Daughters*, she describes how her father kept the real facts about her mother's cancer from both his dying wife and the children. It was only after her mother died that she discovered her father had known for more than a year that her mother was definitely dying. Even though there had been a long illness, there had been no time for anyone except her father to prepare for its inevitable outcome. Only in the final hours of her mother's life, when her condition had deteriorated to a critical point, did Hope Edelman understand fully that her mother was going to die. While she had lived with her mother's illness for a long time, she had never had the information she needed to make sense of it. She had no chance to talk with her mother about what either of them were going through, nor was she able to say goodbye properly. Learning this created considerable problems when it came to mourning. 'The night my mother died,' she writes, 'I entered a survival zone of counterfeit emotions: no tears, no grief, little response at all except a carefully monitored smile and an intense desire to maintain the status quo.'

You can only prepare yourself so much for death. Simply because a parent has been ill does not mean you are necessarily more prepared for their death. Even when there has been plenty of 'warning', death remains unimaginable and largely impossible to prepare for. It is not a shock that can be anticipated, because nothing else that you have ever experienced before is like it. You know it will be dreadful, but before it actually happens you know it with your head rather than your heart.

How you may feel

When someone has died after an illness, the death is a double shock: there is the shock of death itself and there is also the shock of finding yourself still shockable. Your feelings may well contain another shocking emotion: relief. Relief that their agony, and yours, is over. A 12-year-old boy whose mother had suffered from a brain tumour for the last four years was deeply relieved when she finally died. His father's job involved a lot of travel, and he was often alone with his mother overnight, with sole responsibility for looking after her. For four years he had been terrified that she would die while he was there on his own with her. He had endured years of intense anxiety and stress.

As well as relief, another common emotion is anger. You may feel angry that your parent has caused you so much suffering and by dying

41

has taken away any hope for an end to that suffering. The death may even feel like the cause of yet more suffering. Recent research has found that many children who are living with a dying parent experience high levels of anxiety and depression before their parent dies. After their parent dies, they do not feel magically better, but have similar emotions to children bereaved in other ways.[3] A parent's illness may help you prepare in some ways, but at the same time it may simply mean that the arduous process of mourning comes after a period of something equally if differently distressing.

You may be ashamed of these feelings of anger and relief, but they are normal reactions. Remember how as a small child, if you 'lost' your parent in the street or supermarket you became scared and tearful, and then when you found her or him again your reaction was not only relief, but anger too that you were made to feel afraid. It is the same when a parent dies after a long illness: the death brings your fear of loss to an end, and with the end of fear comes rage as well as relief. Perhaps the death also allows you to feel the anger and resentment that it was not possible to express while your parent was still alive, the anger which screams inside you: 'I need you! How dare you get ill! How dare you die! What about me? What about my family? How can you die like this?'

The relief may be for yourself or it may be for your family or for the person who died. You may have longed for your parent to hurry up and die, in which case you may now feel guilty, imagining that your thoughts somehow hastened the end. Or perhaps you feel guilty because you think that while your parent was alive you were sometimes unappreciative.

After a parent dies there is a lot of room for remorse and guilt, a lot of room to regret the things said and not said, the things done and not done. There may be cause for self-recrimination. You may blame yourself for not 'coping better' with the death when you knew it was going to happen. You may blame yourself for not having taken the opportunity while your parent was still alive to say how much you loved him or her. You may blame yourself for your 'weakness' in being scared of what illness has done to your parent.

Jenny remembers racing down the road to a friend's house in a terrified panic one afternoon, sobbing: 'Mum's dying! Mum's dying!' The friend's mother calmed Jenny down a little and went back to the house with her. Upstairs Jenny's mother was lying in bed, screaming with pain, her face a pallid green, the skin tightly drawn across her cheek bones, eyes closed, lips drained of all colour. She was not dead, but she was dying, and she was nearly unconscious with physical pain. For the first time Jenny was seeing all this, seeing fully the nearness and inevitability of death – and understandably enough it terrified her. After her mother's death, however, Jenny felt ashamed that she had not faced death with more self-control and stoicism.

Paul was 17 when his father died of cancer. Years later he still felt guilty that in the final weeks of his father's life he had avoided him, not wanting to touch or be kissed by his father. He remembered in particular one evening when he was passing the door of his father's room. As he passed, his father called out to him to come in and say goodnight. Reluctantly Paul had gone in and hovered at the foot of the bed. 'Come and kiss me goodnight,' his father had said. But Paul could not do it. He did not want to be so near to death, nor to his dying father. He was both frightened and revolted. 'Goodnight,' he said from where he stood and then fled from the room.

For a long time he felt very bad about this cowardice, as he saw it, but gradually over the years Paul, like Jenny, has learnt to be kinder to himself, more realistic about what he could and could not do at the time. Paul can now say to himself, 'Of course I was frightened. Of course I was scared to go near him. I loved him. I loved my father. But I was young and frightened. He was so ill and thin and close to dying. Of course I was scared to go too close.'

For younger children, the feelings of confusion may be still more acute after seeing a parent die after an illness that has altered them physically or emotionally. A boy of 10, whose father had died of cancer, had great difficulty understanding who had actually died. His father had changed dramatically in the course of his illness, putting on a great deal of weight, losing his hair, and becoming prone to abrupt and bizarre mood swings – crying and laughing one moment, whispering, then shouting the next. As Peta Hemmings, the therapist who worked with this child, explained 'James was confronted by a monstrously large man, who neither looked nor sounded like the father who had been playing cricket with him just a few weeks before.' Peta helped this child to come to terms with the difficult truth by playing and talking with him using a special kind of toy. 'It was very painful for him to have to accept that harsh reality, and yet, without that acceptance, the world would have continued to be a very worrying place for him.'

Death after a short illness

Sometimes there will be only a short illness before a parent dies. If your parent died from cancer which was not diagnosed until it was very advanced, or which progressed very rapidly after being detected you will perhaps have more in common with people whose parents have died unexpectedly. This is also so if your parent died after a series of strokes and heart attacks, when the first one does not kill, but leaves the person severely weakened and unable to survive a recurrence. It is also the case if you have been bereaved through accidents which leave a parent fatally hurt. In these situations you will feel both the shocking impact of an unexpected death as well as the anxiety and fear of waiting for death.

When Polly was 21 her mother died suddenly of stomach cancer, after an illness of only two weeks. She had started to have pains in her stomach, and was taken to hospital where doctors diagnosed cancer so advanced that they sent her home for the weekend to be with her family, knowing that it would probably be her last. Polly is one of four sisters. In the last seven days of her mother's life, she, her sisters and her father kept constant vigil at her mother's bedside. It seemed to Polly like years, not days.

Watching the rapid disintegration of the person who in Polly's eyes had always seemed substantial and solid, to someone shrivelled and fragile and wasted, was agonizing. Watching that process take place before her horrified eyes in a matter of days was profoundly disturbing. 'I will never forget how my mother looked in the final days and hours,' she says. 'I will never erase that memory from my mind. I don't think I'll ever get over it and I'm resigned to having to live with it forever.'

The rapid progress of her mother's cancer meant that Polly had both the knowledge that death would happen and the prospect of a future without her mother, as well as the tremendous shock of the unexpectedness of this death. She had to watch the physical decay of her mother over a period of just two weeks, and grapple with the desire to hope and the realization that there was no hope. The one thing that Polly is grateful for is that the illness was sufficiently advanced and death sufficiently inevitable to stop them from 'pretending'. 'I did tell my mother the things I wanted to before she died, that I loved her, and what a wonderful mother she'd been to us. I'm glad we said those things. Perhaps if she'd been ill for longer we would never have got round to it.'

Fifty-five-year-old Martin experienced a number of intensely conflicting emotions both while his 83-year-old father was dying and after his death.

> Dad had been ill with pneumonia for a fortnight and had been in intensive care in hospital. We all thought that was it and it was very gruelling, sitting by his bedside waiting for him to die. Amazingly he pulled through, and ten days later he was discharged. He seemed to have made a complete recovery and was in very good spirits, very pleased to be back home again.

Martin lived two hundred miles from his father and had taken a lot of time off work in order to be with his father at the hospital. He was feeling anxious and resentful about his dual commitments – to his father and to his work.

> I arranged a home help, but I didn't visit him for a week or so after he got home. At some level I suppose I was pretty angry with him for having got better, for having wasted my time. Eventually I arranged to go round, but at the last moment I decided to go to a meeting and catch a later train than plan-ned, so I didn't get there until the evening. I walked in, said hello and sat down in the chair near his bed to have a chat. Almost immediately he started to choke and I guess I just panicked. I was thumping him on the back, and shouting at him, 'Don't die! Don't die!' But he was already unconscious.

Martin's father died in hospital that night, without regaining conscious-ness. Afterwards, Martin struggled with his sense of guilt that he had not made more time to see his father that week, and had arrived so late on the day he died. 'The worst thing was the feeling that as Dad was dying, I'd been shouting at him and hitting him, instead of holding him and telling him I loved him. That memory has just tormented me ever since.'

Sudden death

When a parent dies very unexpectedly, the shock is enormous. Your trust in the world is violated; the foundations of your life are shattered. A sudden death destroys your confidence that life is as you imagine it. Over the years experience teaches us that life is full of loss, that we cannot control the world, that unexpected things will occur and will affect us. Everyone learns this, but usually it is a lesson learned over many years, not in the space of a few minutes. For young people, the shock is especially acute. You are young; you don't expect loss; you are not prepared for it. You may have relatively little experience of loss, still less of the ultimate loss of death. You expect life to be as you see it. Likewise you expect your parents to be *alive*.

A sudden death leaves none of these assumptions and expectations untouched. On the emotional Richter scale, sudden death registers high, and its reverberations are felt a long, long way from the central zone of impact.

Shock is like an illness itself – physical and emotional. People in shock need to stay still, keep warm and rest. After an accident people are often reported to be 'suffering from shock'. The phrase, though used vaguely, describes a specific set of reactions: feeling cold and shivery, confusion, sleeplessness, panic attacks, aches and pains, inability to settle down or concentrate on anything. Emotional shock too can bring on all these reactions and needs the same care and attention. Unfortunately people are not very good at recognizing emotional shock, either in themselves or others. Instead they try to keep busy, distract themselves. Often it takes a more obvious physical illness or an accident to make people realize that they are frail and vulnerable after someone has died. Lily Pincus, in her book *Death and the Family*, describes how she fractured her ankle after her husband's death. While she was being treated, she asked the orthopaedic surgeon if it was common for people to fracture bones after bereavement. Without looking up from her foot, the doctor replied 'Naturally, people lose their sense of balance.'

Violent deaths

One form of bereavement which is particularly hard to come to terms with is when a parent dies not only suddenly, but violently. The experience of children whose parents have been murdered shows beyond doubt the additional weight of rage, anguish and despair that accompanies this kind of loss. Escalating terrorism, rising levels of violent crime, increasing numbers of people travelling by car, train and plane have created a lamentable rise in the number of young people left to face the consequences of a violent death in the family. Post Traumatic Stress Disorder (PTSD) is a term applied to the reaction of surviving victims of plane crashes, bomb attacks, fires, floods and war. It describes the wide range of symptoms suffered in the aftermath of these events, which include nightmares, panic attacks, sweating, shaking, phobias and severe depression. It is a term that applies equally to the bereaved relatives of people killed in tragic and violent ways.

Until comparatively recently it was thought that children did not suffer from any lasting effects of PTSD. However, closer and more detailed studies of children bereaved in violent circumstances have shown that this is simply not the case. In fact, children can experience the same profoundly distressing symptoms as adults. Typically, they will initially be numb and withdrawn, becoming more agitated with time, prone to nightmares, waking fears, flashbacks and behavioural problems, such as bed-wetting or insomnia. Obsessive repetitive habits are also common signs of PTSD. Many of these symptoms, if ignored or treated insensitively, can continue to plague the bereaved child for years.[4]

One girl whose father and brother were killed in the fire at the Bradford football stadium in 1985 still has nightmares about it, and becomes anxious and panicky in enclosed or crowded places. Another young woman whose mother died in the Zeebrugge ferry disaster in 1987 is extremely reluctant to go anywhere near water and suffers from recurring bouts of depression.

When Princess Diana was killed in a car crash in a Paris underpass in August 1997, the entire country seemed to go into mourning. In the months leading up to her death, she had led a high-profile quest for personal happiness and the abrupt and violent ending of her life came as a profound shock to millions of people. The unrelenting tide of details about her death, including photographs of the pulverized car in which she'd been travelling, brought to the attention of many people who would not otherwise have experienced this kind of death the inescapable brutality of it. One can only guess at the anguish suffered by her two sons, Prince William and Prince Harry, as they contemplated what the last moments of their mother's life must have been like. Her physical beauty and vitality in life must have made the wanton devastation of those attributes in death all the more unbearable for them.

As children, we want our parents to protect us from pain, but we want also to protect them. To imagine – to know – that a beloved parent has suffered extreme pain or fear is agony for the child. This is one of the psychological burdens of the bereaved son or daughter *whatever* the cause of death, but when a parent dies in particularly traumatic circumstances that burden is even more intolerable than usual.

Of the various causes of violent death, murder is probably the worst of all and the hardest to come to terms with.

Jake came home one day to find his father had been murdered; it was Jake who found the body. He was 14 at the time. The gratuitousness and viciousness of the attack etched themselves deeply into Jake's being and even in his fifties can still trouble him greatly at times of stress. The images in his mind are hard enough to live with, but the awareness of the proximity of such violence to one's own life is extremely debilitating. How can one trust the world when such horrific things happen? How is one to believe that life is worth living? The combination of suspicion, uncertainty and terror caused by this kind of death is very real and takes time and often professional help to learn to live with.

Every year in the UK at least fifty children endure the trauma of one of their parents killing the other. In the USA more women are murdered by husbands or partners than are killed in car accidents or by unknown attackers. The children who find themselves orphaned in this way have often witnessed their parent's murder and, even if spared that horror, their lives are invariably plunged into disarray. They have to leave their homes, often with no chance to take precious toys or possessions. They may find themselves living with relations they hardly know, many miles from where they lived before. They may find themselves living temporarily in children's homes or with foster families. The uncertainty and unfamiliarity of their living arrangements is an extreme additional pressure on children already traumatized by the violent death of one parent and the abrupt loss of another. In addition these children may have already endured or witnessed years of horrific domestic violence. All the difficulties that children bereaved in less extreme ways so often experience as a result of adults failing to inform, consult or listen are vastly compounded for children who lose a parent in violent circumstances. What they urgently need is clear information; space and time to go over what has happened to them; caring and supportive adults who can listen to their fears and contain their anxieties without censoring or judging, and, in most cases, professional help by psychiatrists specially trained to work with children bereaved of one parent by the other. Above all they need sensitive and effective support to process their trauma.

Without proper support, the devastating impact of violent deaths can last a lifetime. Two people I know whose parents died in violent circumstances – in both cases the victims of terrorist attacks, one in Northern Ireland, the other in Beirut – still bear deep emotional and psychological scars. Neither has recovered confidence and trust in the world, and neither lives anything like a fulfilling life, even though their respective parents died more than ten years ago. For them, the feelings of fear, anger and desolation which are normal after a parent's death, are magnified to vast and crippling proportions.

But terrible as it is, violent death need *not* be a permanently devastating experience for the bereaved. People can and do recover with time, often with the help of a skilled therapist or counsellor. The Royal Free Hospital in London runs a special clinic for children and adolescents who have suffered the acute psychological trauma of one parent murdering the other. Since 1986, the psychiatrists at the Royal Free have seen hundreds of children from such families. A follow-up survey from the clinic showed that skilled support after a loss of this kind made a significant difference to the individual's ability to recover from his or her experience.

This was the case for Richard, a 21-year-old who came to the Stress Clinic. His brother was killed when a party boat sank on the River Thames in 1989 after colliding with another boat. Richard found it very consoling to meet and talk with other young people in similar situations who understood how he was feeling and what he was going through.

The urgent need to blame, the sense of rage at the world, the lack of trust in everything around you – all these are natural reactions to a harrowing event. To lose a parent in this way is shocking beyond belief, and the after-effects of such trauma are themselves shocking and painful. It is well known that many of the children of people murdered in the Nazi concentration camps in the Second World War, even though they may not have been in camps themselves (and even though they are now adults with children and grandchildren of their own), have continued to suffer emotionally and psychologically as a result of the terrible way in which their parents died.

Whether you are part of a community of sufferers, like Richard, or suffering in isolation, like Jake, makes little difference to how you come to terms with your grief. Knowing other people are in the same situation can only help if you are able to *talk* about your shared experience and derive some sense of meaning from it. Holocaust survivors and their children tended for a long time after World War II to avoid discussing and sharing memories of their trauma, anger and grief, wishing instead to hide from their sense of shame and guilt and escape the stigma of the past. Understandable as this reaction is, it does not in the long term help people to assimilate their experiences, or come to terms with their grief.

By contrast, many of the children who lost parents in the attacks on the World Trade Centre in New York on 11th September 2001 seem to have been helped by the worldwide sympathy for their loss and condemnation of the attacks themselves. Over 3,000 children under the age of 18 lost a parent in the attacks. Some were babies, the average age was 9. Some of their parents were firefighters, others were working in the offices of the World Trade Centre, others were passengers on the hijacked planes. Fifteen-year-old Madison Burnett was 5 when her father died on the third plane aimed that same day at the White House in Washington, a plan he helped to thwart. As she told the *Independent* newspaper ten years on:

> We were all in the sitting room and mum got a phone call and I remember her crying hysterically, but she wouldn't tell us what was wrong. What we didn't know was that it was my dad, phoning to say that he was on board a hi-jacked plane. She turned on the TV and we could see these buildings falling down. It was all really crazy. I just remember the sound of my mum crying, and staring in horror at the images on the TV. Most of the rest of the day is a blank, although what I do remember is looking out of the window when it was dark, and seeing that our neighbours had formed a human chain around our home, to stop the TV cameramen and journalists getting near to us. And that was when my Mum told us that Dad had died, that he wouldn't be coming back. It's very difficult to think of anything positive that comes of losing a parent like this, but I do try to think about what I've learned. I think it's so important to talk, to

explore how you feel. I have lots of good memories of my
dad: he was so warm, and he loved us so much. And, of
course, I'm proud of him too, and of what he did on board
the flight.[5]

Caitlin Langone was 12 when her father, a firefighter, died.

He'd been in lots of dangerous places before and he'd always
come home. Over the next few days my brother and I carried
on going to school and things seemed normal, so I was still
sure things would be OK. It was only when it got to a week after
the attack that I started getting unsure. But in a way I was
numb to it – it was simply too big a thing to contemplate, that he
might never be coming back. In a way the biggest consolation
I have [is] that he at least died doing the job he loved. And
I guess it's a help that he was there as a firefighter, that he was
dedicated to what he did and that he was prepared to die to save
others. That makes his death maybe easier to accept. He died
being the best person he could possibly have been, and that's
pretty special.[6]

For children whose parents were simply in the wrong place at the
wrong time, making sense of their death has been harder. Thea Trinidad
was 10 when her father died in his office on the 103rd floor of one of the
twin towers.

The thing I've found hard to live with, through the years, is the
thought that my dad's death was planned – that it was a murder,
and the murderers plotted for so long, and that they cared so
little for the people whose lives they were going to take, or their
families. I don't hate people because they're a certain religion or
from a certain part of the world, but I hate the people who were
involved.[7]

Dr Gary Jackson, a psychiatrist at the Middlesex Hospital in London,
works with people bereaved in traumatic circumstances. 'People tend to
fantasize about the death,' he says. 'They wonder what the last moments
were like, how terrifying it was, whether they [the victim] were in pain.
Then they may feel intensely guilty about these morbid preoccupations
which are in fact an important part of accepting what has happened.'

According to Dr Jackson, there can also be an intense need to blame, in
the often urgent attempt to find a reason, an explanation, for the death.

This can be helpful, as long as it does not become a way of avoiding your own feelings of loss. Most important of all, for anyone coping with a bereavement and especially for those whose parents have died in unnatural circumstances, is *talking*. It is, says Dr Jackson, 'the single most significant factor' in how well people adjust and recover. 'It doesn't take away the pain, but talking is enormously beneficial.'[8]

Violent deaths of all kinds are extremely hard to accept and come to terms with. They can have a very damaging effect on the way you see yourself, the way you see the world and the way you feel about life in general. If you are struggling in the aftermath of this kind of bereavement, you should not try to 'go it alone'. It will be far more helpful for you to find someone to talk to, whether a relative, a friend, a priest or a counsellor. The advantage of a trained counsellor or therapist is that they will know how to 'hear' what you are saying, they will in all likelihood (and you should check this) have experience of listening to other people who've been through similar experiences, and will understand and accept what you are going through, not be shocked, or tell you to 'get over it'. If you can talk to someone in this way, it will help enormously in coming to terms with your experience.

Death by suicide

Suicide is undoubtedly one of the most difficult kinds of bereavement to come to terms with. When a parent kills himself or herself it can leave you with deep feelings of guilt, resentment, anger, helplessness and inadequacy. The stigma attached to suicide makes things still more difficult as it is not so easy to talk about what happened and the sense of shame is especially painful: instead of rousing extra compassion in friends and relatives, as might be expected, the idea that something shocking and desperate has happened can, tragically, often work the other way and create a wall of silence between you and the world. This sense of isolation, not only outside your family but within it too, is an additional source of distress and unhappiness for many young people.[9]

In America, death by suicide is now the fourth most common cause of death before the age of 49, and between 10,000 and 60,000 children and teenagers are estimated to lose a parent by suicide in America each year.[10] In Europe, deaths by suicide have increased by 60 per cent in the past fifty years, and in Northern Ireland, is now one of the leading causes of premature death.[11] A number of studies have found, unsurprisingly, that young people bereaved in this way experience higher levels of shame and anger and have more difficulty accepting their parent's death than children bereaved in other ways. Not all children bereaved by suicide will have particular problems afterwards by any means, but with suicide, it is not just the death itself, but what came before and what happens after that can make grieving that much harder.[12]

A group of children in Northern Ireland, who took part in a two day residential programme for families bereaved by suicide, found it a huge relief to be able to speak openly, without shame about what had happened to them.[13] Aged between 8 and 16, all the children who attended the weekend wanted to know more about suicide in general as well as needing to tell their own story without fear of rejection. Doing so helped them to feel less guilty and confused about their parent's death. One girl who'd been unable to tell people how her father had died before the weekend, felt confident enough to do so afterwards. Others found it easier to talk about their feelings and worries to their remaining parent, as well as finding themselves better able to understand their parent's emotions. 'I understand why mammy feels angry', one child said. Another found that the weekend helped her to realize that 'Daddy would want us to be happy again. He wouldn't think bad of us for being happy.'

As well as the sense of shame that people bereaved by suicide often feel, the sense that something disgraceful and, literally, unspeakable has occurred, feelings of intense guilt often come with this kind of bereavement. You may believe that you should or could have done something to prevent the death. You may feel considerable anger towards the person who has died, towards other people for not having done more to prevent the death, and towards yourself.

Mary's father killed himself when she was 15. Her parents' marriage had been turbulent and they had divorced two years earlier. Her father had subsequently become very depressed. After his death, a well-meaning relation told Mary that before he died her father had said that he felt he'd failed his children and that they no longer loved him. Mary interpreted this as meaning that if she had made more effort to show her father that she loved him, he would not have killed himself. For over ten years the belief that she was to blame for his death was a terrible secret that Mary carried inside her. It was not until she went for counselling in her late twenties that she was able to admit to another person that she held herself responsible for her father's suicide. The simple act of telling someone else came as a great relief. With the counsellor, Mary then began to explore her feelings about her father's death for the first time. By facing the deep and frightening belief that she was to blame, Mary began to discover how unfounded her sense of guilt was.

Perhaps the greatest problem for people trying to come to terms with this kind of death is the legacy of fear that it leaves behind. There is often a deeply-held belief and fear that you too will be the victim of self-destructive impulses. It is not at all uncommon for people coping with a death by suicide to become preoccupied with suicide themselves. In fact, thinking about suicide is very common after a parent has taken their own life. You may feel doomed or fated to the same end. I have heard it said of the family of a friend whose mother committed suicide: 'There is bad blood on the mother's side. She was not the first. They all have it in them.' 'It' being the capacity to take their own lives.

This kind of myth-making is dangerous and foolish and incorrect. Whether it comes from you or from other people, it is immensely distressing. The particularly intense helplessness you feel after someone you love has committed suicide can make you feel as if you have no control whatsoever over yourself. Everyone has this experience to some degree after a death, but it is the circumstances of a suicide and society's reaction to it, as well as the complicated nature of your own reaction, that gives this idea of being doomed so much force. Thinking about suicide is common – part of the way the human brain processes traumatic events is to replay them and ruminate on them. But to believe that anyone is fated to kill themselves is simply wrong. Suicide is not written in the stars or genetically inherited; it is a personal choice that a person makes, whether for rational or irrational reasons.

Gary is now in his thirties. His father committed suicide when he was a child. The tragedy of this talented and popular man's death, the violence and the shame of it, silenced the whole family. What could be said about such a dreadful thing? Their own sense of shame, guilt and anger, and the embarrassment of others, deepened this silence until it became an impenetrable wall around each of them, and between them and the world. Gary was 21 when he met an old friend of his father's. Until then, he had never talked to anyone about his father's death. The friend knew far more about his father and about his father's death than Gary did himself, and was pleased to share his memories with Gary. He had not even known until then how his father had killed himself, let alone where and why. It came as a tremendous relief to discover some of the basic facts about his father's life and death, and this enabled him to grieve at last.

You *need* to know the facts after a suicide. The more information you have the less room there is for myth-making and the many problems it causes.[14] There is enough darkness already: where you can shed light on this terrible event, it is important to do so.

Suicide does not usually happen suddenly in a single act of violence. Often people who take their own lives will have struggled with mental health problems for a long time beforehand. There may have been earlier, unsuccessful suicide attempts. The stress of living with a parent with severe depression, mood disorders or other psychiatric conditions is very real and takes its toll on every person in the family. Children whose parents kill themselves will often have had to cope with a chaotic family life in the years or months leading up to the death: unpredictable behaviour, high levels of domestic and marital conflict, financial difficulties and legal problems, and divorce are all more common in families in which a parent kills him or herself than in other bereaved households. The impact of living with this kind of strain over a long period of time *before* your parent died is something that puts you more at risk after the death, and these distressing aspects of your experience also need to be taken into account.[15]

Sometimes people will kill themselves systematically over an extended period of time, as is the case for people who die from alcohol or drug abuse. Although these kinds of death are not seen as suicide, if your parent died in this way the feelings you may have about the death are very much akin to those experienced by people who have been bereaved by a suicide, with all the extreme complexity that involves.

Sally, now in her forties, was 26 when her mother killed herself by jumping in front of a train in the London Underground. There was the horror of imagining what had been done to her mother physically when the train hit her. There was the horror of imagining what had been going through her mother's mind at the time. There was the anguish of the daughter whose mother not only destroyed her own life, but also through that act somehow attacked Sally's right to be alive. But although her mother's death was a shock, it was not entirely unexpected. As long as she could remember her mother had been very disturbed. She had distinct memories from childhood of her mother becoming hysterical and, finally, of the day when an ambulance arrived at the house and her mother was taken away and committed to a psychiatric hospital. She had tried to kill herself before. The difference was that this time she was successful. For Sally the damage of her mother's despair had been done before she died. Sally had been suffering since she was a child. She had felt many of the feelings that come after a suicide, while her mother was still alive.

Rachel's mother died from liver failure two days after Rachel's twenty-third birthday. She had been a chronic alcoholic for almost as long as Rachel could remember. It had been years since they had been able to hold a coherent conversation, and in the past twelve months her mother had no longer been able to recognize her when she visited. Watching this kind of self-destruction was immensely painful. Seeing her mother drunk and often violent was terribly upsetting. Witnessing this, helpless to do anything to stop it, Rachel felt guilty, ashamed, angry, wretched – and, to protect herself, finally managed to stop feeling very much at all. When her mother finally died, it was a relief, but it also stirred up all the emotions she had protected herself from over the years. The death she had somehow to mourn was complicated: it was both a suicide and a death after a long illness. Her grief was also complicated and drawn out.

At a profound and often unconscious level, a parent's suicide can seem like a personal rejection and this is something that often haunts children whose parents have died in this way. In reality, what your parent was rejecting was not you, but the misery of living with their own anguish, pain and despair. For people sunk in the depths of severe depression or suffering from an incurable illness, the feeling of letting their children down, of being a failure as a parent, can seem so unbearable that they may even persuade themselves they are removing themselves to help and protect you. Rejecting you was probably the very last thing your parent was thinking, and yet this feeling of personal rejection is still intensely painful and extremely difficult to live with.

John was 18 when his mother killed herself. Despite the fact that she had a history of severe depression, he felt that he was somehow to blame for her death. Years afterwards he still carried with him the fear that she had rejected him because of some failure on his part, and this powerful emotional cocktail of self-blame and fear of rejection made it extremely difficult for John to recover from his mother's death and move on in his own life. Whenever he got close to someone, he became terrified that sooner or later she too would reject him. To protect himself from this, he would become highly critical and destructive, thus preventing the relationship from developing. It was not until this pattern of behaviour had been going on for several years that John sought the help of a therapist and came to see how his unresolved feelings about his mother's suicide were making it impossible for him to trust anyone else.

Anita, now 25, also blamed herself for her father's death, even though she was only 13 when he killed himself. She too felt profoundly rejected by his death, and increasingly anxious to avoid ever experiencing similar feelings of rejection. At home she tried to be the perfect daughter, always helpful and good-tempered; at school she worked very hard, was endlessly supportive to friends, and never allowed herself to show any feelings of irritation, anger or despair. It was as if she took on more and more responsibility for other people's wellbeing to compensate for her earlier failure – as she saw it – to make her father happy. But behind the facade, Anita's buried fears were growing, not fading: several years after her father's death, with the additional pressure of exams, she found she could no longer control her anxiety and began to suffer frequent panic attacks. It was only then that she began to look at the legacy of her father's suicide and to see how it was damaging her.

It is important to realize that by the time people have reached the stage where they are able to kill themselves, they are so sunk down in their own unhappiness that their sense of reality has become distorted, and their way of thinking profoundly affected. No one becomes suicidal overnight, and what one individual says or does is rarely enough to save a person's life when he or she is intent on taking it. It is the accumulation of many, many things, not one single event or individual, that drives someone to such despair. To imagine a person you love in such distress is heart-breaking, but you are not responsible for their despair, nor for the problems behind it, nor for their decision to end their lives.

How you may feel

When a parent dies very unexpectedly it comes as a tremendous shock. You may feel very agitated and restless in the first few days. The shock and the sense of being in danger and of being suddenly very vulnerable, bring on a rush of adrenalin. In former times people might have needed this adrenalin for 'fight or flight', but nowadays, following a death, they sit around with family and friends drinking endless cups of tea, and there is no practical need for the adrenalin racing through their systems. You want to *do* something, but with death there is nothing to be done. You want to run and hide, but there is nowhere to go. The thing you most want to avoid is no longer avoidable. Neither fight nor flight are any use to you. This useless adrenalin may make you feel slightly sick and light-headed at first.

Fixation on a seemingly irrelevant or insignificant detail is another common reaction to the shock of a death, and not an indication of lack of feeling. You might feel afraid to cross the road, anxious if relations go on holiday, hyper-aware of the possibility of train or car crashes. These are normal preoccupations when you are trying to take on board the enormous shock of a sudden death. Shock makes people behave in very strange ways, when viewed in the cool calm light of rationality. But at the time, there is no rationality, no normality. Your body takes over in order to give your mind a chance to take in this staggering information.

Shirley's mother died of a heart attack when Shirley was 24. They were very close and Shirley was devastated by her death. On the day of the funeral, she recalls, she could think of nothing but what she should wear. 'Several people were quite disapproving. They thought I was being cal-lous, fussing about my dress, but it wasn't that, it was just a way of coping with the awfulness of it all. Fixing my mind on something that was still there and real.'

James had been on his way to the bank when the news arrived that his father had died. Not knowing what else to do, James continued as planned – though he cannot now remember arriving at the bank, or leaving it again.

Later on, as the shock begins to wear off, your mind may take over again, sometimes leaving you furiously angry or frightened or depressed. These are the feelings that shock protected you from.

Jeremy, 19 when his mother died of a heart attack, seemed fine at first, coping with everything, organizing everything, managing everything. It was only after a few months had passed, and his body had switched off the red alert button, that he began to feel all the emotions that until then he had held at bay. He became depressed and prone to outbursts of temper. He also started to drink heavily. Gradually he was able to connect his feelings and behaviour with his mother's death, and see how the shock of her death had been so great at the time that it had inured him to the pain of grief. Now the shock had worn off, but the pain was there still and had to be lived through.

As the days and weeks pass you may also find yourself feeling guilty, thinking that you could have done something to prevent the death, or that things you did somehow caused it. 'If only,' you say. 'If only I'd been quieter, nicer, less selfish, less difficult. If only I'd come home earlier that evening. If only I hadn't had that fight with my brother.' The list of 'if onlys' is endless, but usually guilt is irrational. Ask yourself what, realistically, you could have done or not done, and you will probably find the answer comes back as 'not much'. It is not possible to lead your life as if people are about to die any moment, and you shouldn't now start expecting yourself to, or berating yourself for not having done so.

Sometimes after a sudden death, particularly when it is part of a larger catastrophe involving many other people, there is a powerful need to blame. If only someone can be blamed, you think, then maybe you can make some sense of this death and make sure such a thing doesn't happen again. But it is important to understand that even where there is genuine cause for finger-pointing, the underlying need is to diminish your own personal feeling of being horribly powerless.

Helplessness

To protect yourself from what can become an obsessional desire to blame, you need to understand why the acute feelings of helplessness after a sudden death are so painful and bewildering. Feeling helpless threatens your fundamental sense of purpose, usefulness and significance in the world. Shakespeare puts this feeling of overwhelming meaninglessness into words in his play, *Hamlet,* when the young prince says:

> O! that this too, too solid flesh would melt,
> Thaw and resolve itself into a dew ...
> How weary, stale, flat and unprofitable
> Seem to me all the uses of this world!

Suddenly the world seems nothing more than a 'quintessence of dust'. You find you are no more significant or powerful than a bit of rubbish in the sea, pulled back and forth and tossed about without any say in the matter. For teenagers, in particular, it is especially hard to feel so helpless at a time in your life when you expected to be taking control of your life, not losing control.

Feeling helpless is very painful, but it doesn't last. You are not responsible for everything that happens in your life, but neither are you entirely out of control of events. Accepting that you could do nothing to prevent your parent's death is hard but vital. One of the major tasks we face in life is learning when we can take charge and when we can't. Charles Dickens' story, *A Christmas Carol,* is about a man who thinks he can control life, but learns through a little crippled boy and a few ghostly visitors that he is not so much in control as he likes to think. And when it comes to death, he learns, he has no control whatsoever. Through this realization, however, he learns that he does have control in other areas of his life, and is motivated from then on to put his energy and time to better use than he has before.

Anger

Feelings of helplessness can often turn to feelings of intense anger and you may find yourself thinking furious thoughts about your dead parent, your family, the world: How dare this happen! How dare life deal this card! How dare people die like this! How dare the world conspire to hurt me this way!

Rage and helplessness are two sides of the same coin. Rage is often easier to bear, however, and perhaps the hardest thing to believe right now is that to be able to grieve you must also *allow* yourself to feel helpless. Feeling the pain of loss is a key aspect of grieving for a dead parent, however unpleasant and frightening. You have to stop trying to pin the blame on yourself or anyone else; you have to stop imagining you can protect yourself from ever again experiencing such pain as this; you have to feel this awful helplessness for a while, because it is only by letting go of responsibility for the event and letting go of the need to be in control, that you can begin to put death into some perspective which in turn allows you to mourn your loss and live your life.

Accidents and illness

Bereavement is one of the greatest causes of stress in a person's life, and stress weakens the immune system, so it's not too surprising that people of all ages are more susceptible to illnesses and accidents after a parent's death. It is well recognized that a major shock can bring on an underlying illness, or trigger illness. Physical illness can also be a response to stress, or it can be a way to express stress or unhappiness. There is clear evidence from many different countries and cultures that being bereaved of a close relative increases your own risk of illness, especially when the death is sudden.[16]

Bereaved children of all ages are vulnerable to physical illness and accident after a major loss. One in five children in the Childhood Bereavement Study, for example, had frequent headaches for the first time in the first few months after their parent died, and for some these symptoms of grief and stress continued into the second year, especially amongst girls.[17] Children in families where the death was followed by a lot of disruption and change were found to be most likely to be suffering from a range of physical ailments, and illness was most common in children who'd lost fathers. Serious illness after a parent dies is less usual, but amongst the children in the Childhood Bereavement Study, rates of serious illness rose from 4 per cent to 10 per cent in the first year after a parent's death, and were far higher than in non-bereaved children of the same age.[18]

Accidents are also more common in the months after a parent's death, especially amongst boys. While the death of a father seems to make children more vulnerable to illness, the death of a mother seems to increase the likelihood of accident. One in four children in the Childhood Bereavement Study had accidents in the early months after a death, the majority of them teenaged boys. Nearly half of the teenage boys in the study had accidents during the first year after their parent had died, often bad enough to require medical attention. When the researchers looked in more depth at why some children had accidents and others didn't, the researchers found that those who had accidents were anxious, felt personally unsafe, and were showing disturbed behaviour in other ways, such as social withdrawal, attention-seeking, aggressive and delinquent behaviour.[19] It's not only that bereavement can quite literally knock you off balance for a while. For children and teenagers, it's also often easier to express difficult and painful emotions through physical symptoms. Getting hurt may be a way to show that you are feeling hurt. Being unsafe may be a way to show that you are feeling unsafe. For children who feel guilty and in some way to blame for their parent's death, physical pain may be a way of expressing a belief that they deserve to feel pain. Or it may be a veiled cry for help, a way of asking for the attention and care they badly need but are not getting from the adults around them. Another explanation for the increased risk of illness and accident in children after parents die is that it is caused by an unconscious desire to bring back the parent who has died to care for them.

Loose ends

With a sudden death, there are also likely to be lots of loose ends. Finances and personal affairs may be in considerable disorder. Both my father and stepfather died intestate – without making wills. Both had a number of debts. Neither of them had life insurance policies or even owned their own homes. Sorting these things out can often fall to you as an older child, and may make you see your dead parent in a new light, and not necessarily a very nice one.

Peter was 23 when his father died suddenly and he had to help his mother sort through his father's affairs. Not only did Peter find considerable chaos in his father's financial business – bills long overdue, debts his mother had not known about – he also came across love letters from another woman. It seemed his father had been leading a double life for years. Peter needed to alter his view of his father as a reliable family-loving man. To discover this new man at a time when he was still deeply shaken by the sudden loss of the old one was shattering. It took a long time for Peter to adjust his view and see not only the father who had indeed been devoted and loving, but also the man who had been disorganized and dishonest. Forgiving his father for being this less likeable person was made harder because of not being able to discuss it with him. Peter felt very angry towards his father for a long time, for deceiving them all and for adding this extra hurt to the pain of his death. It was several years before he could fully accept the man his father was and accept that his love and his anger did not cancel each other out, but could exist alongside each other.

Death can also be a time of concealment as well as disclosure.

Ian's mother asked him to go and collect the results of the post mortem after his father's sudden death. The report showed not only heart disease but also cirrhosis of the liver, caused by his father's heavy but largely secret drinking. In the last few years his father had gone to considerable lengths to hide his drinking from his wife. Ian had to decide whether or not it was necessary to tell his mother the full details of the report. In the end he decided not to, but making this decision meant taking responsibility for the undisclosed information. At 21 that was not an easy burden to shoulder.

Other kinds of death

Sometimes you may feel you have already lost your parent *before* the actual death. A parent may have 'died' already, for example, following a stroke or illness such as multiple sclerosis, as both can change the personality completely. These changes in your parent before death may have been so great that you felt as if you had lost the person you loved months or years before the eventual 'real' death: the irritable, dependent, silent person is not the mother or father you knew. A stroke or heart attack can literally kill the parent you knew, leaving behind a very changed person. As E.E. Cummings put it, 'unbeing dead isn't being alive'.

In situations like these, you may have had to mourn for the loss of a parent before the death itself, and this can make it very hard to know precisely what you have lost *after* the death. You may find that you have been living in a kind of limbo which the death brings to an end and that only then may the pent-up feelings of sadness, fear, rage and guilt be released. To feel these emotions after a period of suspended animation can be a tremendous shock if you had mistakenly believed the numbness was a genuine ability to cope calmly with what was happening. When your parent dies in some sense and yet lives on in another, it can be very hard to mourn properly for what you have lost. You may feel unentitled to be sad, or you may feel relieved that your parent has died at last. In Orthodox Jewish communities this death-in-life is recognized formally: when a person narrowly escapes death, whether through illness or accident, they can if they wish change their name, i.e. they can assume a new identity and start a new life. This tradition recognizes that you cannot come close to death and *not* lose part of yourself: when you are touched by death, a part of you dies, even if you survive.

Another way in which you can lose a parent before they have actually died is when your parents are separated or divorced. This increasingly common scenario can add significantly to the already complicated mix of emotions after a parent's death.

Gina's parents divorced when she was 5, after which she spent the term times with her mother and the holidays with her father. 'I had a complicated relationship with my father,' Gina explains. 'In some ways he was a difficult man to know, and of course I didn't see that much of him. There were a lot of things left unsaid when he died, unaired grievances as well as unexpressed affection.' Gina found it hard to know where to begin mourning for her father. Anger and resentment, pain, love and sorrow all crowded in on her in a great bewildering muddle. Eventually she decided to go to a psychotherapist to try to sort out her feelings about his death. 'After a year of thinking and talking and crying I began to feel I was getting somewhere, beginning to understand what his death meant to me and how to cope with it.' What Gina also began to understand was that in many ways her father's death was just the icing on the cake. Underneath lay a great many other feelings – equally tormented and tangled – about her parents' divorce.

> I started to realize that I had 'lost' my father long before he died. I had lost him when I was a little girl, when he was no longer there to pick me up from school, meet my teachers, watch me on sports day, admire my paintings, criticize my clothes, disapprove of my boyfriends, dig into his pocket for loose change, grumble when I came home late or congratulate me on my successes. All the normal everyday things a father is to a daughter were not part of our relationship, and I had a lot of mourning to catch up on for all those things I had lost.

With the help of a therapist, Gina began to see how important it was to recognize that she had lost her father *before* he died, in order to understand fully the meaning of his physical death. The two losses had to be separated before she could fit them together again in a way that made sense.

Karen is in a similar position: her mother remarried a few years ago when Karen was 16 and although both her parents are still alive, her mother's new husband will not let Karen see her mother at all. Their relationship has to be conducted by telephone when the stepfather is out. Recently her mother invited Karen and her boyfriend to lunch. Thinking and hoping that perhaps the situation had changed, they drove over to the house, but when they got there, Karen's stepfather had locked every single door in the house and was standing outside the front door waving the keys, brandishing his fist. Karen is grappling with how to grieve for her mother while her mother is still alive. She can see what she has lost and can even admit how like a death it is. 'In some ways it would be easier if she *were* dead,' Karen says. 'She might as well be, but she isn't. It makes it really hard. I am so angry about it – and I miss her so much. But then she's still alive, so what am I supposed to do?'

It is very common for children of divorced or separated parents to lose all contact with the parent they no longer live with. This may happen gradually after one or other parent moves away from the area, or it may happen rapidly, perhaps as a result of hostility between the parents or because the parent thinks it is in the children's best interest. Whatever the cause, the reasons are seldom thought out or explained, and the children are left with a bitter legacy of bewilderment, despair, guilt and anger. They feel profoundly rejected, but also confused about their role in the rejection. Were they to blame in some way? Had they done something wrong? Worse still, were they intrinsically unlovable? Why did their parent no longer want to see them, know them, love them?

Whether through divorce or death, losing a parent in childhood is linked to a greater risk of psychological problems, such as depression and anxiety, in adulthood. In a recent British study of 50 adults who were brought up in stepfamilies, both those who lost a parent through death and those who lost a parent through marital breakdown experienced difficulties that were often long lasting.[20] The children whose parents had divorced were less likely to have psychological problems as adults, but twice as likely to have serious difficulties in their relationships. Both groups had been deeply frightened and confused as children by their parent's disappearance, and not given the emotional support and information they needed. One woman who was 7 when her mother left the family described how she had been 'petrified' and had clung to her father, screaming when he had to leave the house to go to work. Nightmares, bed-wetting, school phobia were all typical symptoms of these children's feelings of insecurity. In the majority of cases, no one had explained to them what was happening, or else they had been given dishonest or misleading explanations. Children whose parents had divorced or separated in many ways had a more difficult time coming to terms with their loss than those who had died. First, they had often endured years of conflict, discord and sometimes violence in their family; second, the reasons for their parent's absence were less explicable than if the parent had died; third, they tended to have more negative feelings towards their absent parent. Nevertheless, what comes through most clearly from this research are the *similarities* in the experiences of these children. While society may react differently to divorce and death, as far as the grieving child is concerned the loss of a parent in childhood is nearly always an unparalleled disaster whatever the reason. For both groups of children, their loss was augmented by the strain of the disruption to their home life, the struggle to comprehend what was happening to them, and, sooner or later, the arrival of stepparents and stepsiblings.

In 1990, Neti-Neti Theatre Company developed and staged a play about loss and bereavement among young people. The play is called simply *Grief* and is about the sudden death of a teenager and the effect his death has on his sister and their friends. One of the teenagers is Hazel, whose mother has walked out on the family. Eddie's death arouses Hazel's memories and feelings of loss about her mother.

> [Dad] locked himself in the bathroom for an hour. Later he got drunk and burnt all her things. I had to grow up overnight … She never did come back, but we carried on. It was like a pantomime for all the family.

Later Hazel finds a photograph of her mother and brings it out at teatime. 'Where did you find that?' her father demands. She replies:

> Buried in a cupboard. She's not dead as far as I know. She was a bright, ordinary woman who'd had enough. As I remember. And I for one don't intend to forget her. *[She puts the photo down in front of her mother's empty chair and says to the audience:]* Any loss is a bereavement, not just death.

To put it another way, there are many kinds of death, not just the cessation of life. Mourning a lost parent is very difficult to do while they are still alive in some form or some place. And when that parent does eventually die in the conventional sense of the word, the process of grieving for them will be greatly complicated, for you will need to mourn both the person you lost in life and the person you have lost through death.

Coping with guilt

However a parent died, one of the most troubling emotions the death can leave you with is guilt. Young children are very vulnerable to feelings of guilt as they tend to believe they are somehow responsible for the death. This is called 'magical thinking' and is a back-to-front way of dealing with the terrible sense of helplessness that so often accompanies the death of a loved one. The belief that one somehow caused the death, for the young child creates the possibility that they might somehow be able to reverse it. It is a way of denying the finality of death, which for young children, is so difficult to understand. If you believe you somehow caused Mummy to disappear, there may be some as yet undiscovered way of making her appear again. This is why young children particularly need clear, consistent and honest information about their parent's death, and why vague explanations about 'going to live with Jesus', or vague phrases such as 'passing on', are unhelpful and confusing, leaving room for the child to invent explanations that may be soothing in the short term, but can create serious problems with low-self-esteem, anxiety and fearfulness in the long term. A child of 6 who believes she caused her father to die by being naughty may internalize that belief and in her adult relationships suppress her own needs and feelings out of unconscious fear she will again drive a loved one away. Allowing young children to express their sense of guilt and helping them to realize they are not responsible for their parent's death is, thus, hugely important. But because it never occurs to the adults around them to think the child blames him or herself, this kind of help often gets missed.

But whatever your age, blaming yourself, regretting things you said or did, wishing you had done things differently, are all part of the package of guilt that can land so heavily in your lap after a parent's death. These feelings of guilt and remorse and self-recrimination need to be looked at, calmly and kindly. You may have grounds for some regret or remorse, but hating yourself for what you did or didn't do will not help you. It is far better to try to understand why you behaved as you did and accept that it has happened now. It is done. Try to understand and accept, rather than judge and accuse.

After my father died I felt particularly guilty about the fact that I had avoided going to see him the year he died. Holidays were precious and I wanted the time to be out with my boyfriend and friends, not bored and lonely staying with my Dad. After my father died I found a letter from him, sent a month or two before, asking me to come and spend at least part of the summer holidays with him. 'I've only seen you for two days this year,' he had written. 'Is a week or two too much to ask?' Evidently it was, because I managed to evade the trip north to stay with him and in fact saw him only once more, for a weekend in London, before he died.

I felt guilty, *awful*, about that for a long time, about how I must have hurt him by not wanting to visit, not caring that I hadn't seen him all year. He must have thought I didn't love him. And now I would never be able to tell him, or show him, or in any way let him know. Maybe he had died thinking his only daughter did not love him. How could I live with that?

Now I try and tell myself that he was a grown man, that probably he understood that at 17, friends seem more important than parents, that it was more fun for me being with my friends than with him. I hope he understood. It is still a matter of deep regret to me that I was not more interested in my father in those last years of his life. I would have liked to have known him a little better than I do. But I am able now to tell myself that my behaviour was not so reprehensible, it was normal for a 17-year-old; that I am not to blame for his death nor the timing of it; that neither of us could have known time was so limited; that hopefully he knew I loved him.

The guilt you may feel is usually not deserved nor the cause of it as significant as you may imagine. Your parent will have understood that you were frightened by his or her illness and impending death, and long ago forgiven a moment's irritation, a cross word, a brusque gesture, a refusal to help, a cruel phrase flung out in anger. You must forgive yourself these things too – remember how understandable in the circumstances your behaviour was; allow yourself to remember the moments when you *were* there, *did* listen, *did* care, *did* help. You are not a saint or an angel. No one in the world – except you at this moment – either expects or expected you to be.

Everyone experiences some guilt after someone they care for dies, whoever that person was and however they died. 'If only I'd been more supportive, spent more time with her,' one 24-year-old was still saying five years later about his friend who committed suicide at university. 'Why didn't I go and see him off at the station. I didn't even kiss him goodbye,' a woman says about her husband who died of a heart attack the next day. 'Why did we have that stupid argument that morning?' asks a 21-year-old, whose fiancé was killed that afternoon in a climbing accident.

What you are asking yourself is why you are mortal: why you aren't a superhuman being who can foresee these tragedies, predict the future and act accordingly. People often torment themselves in the months and years after a person's death with these regrets, whether that person died slowly or suddenly, calmly or violently, while asleep or in an accident. The regrets will differ with the circumstances of the death, but everyone is susceptible to feelings of guilt and blame. But feeling guilty will not do any good, least of all to yourself. You can't live your life as if it will end at lunchtime. You have to assume life will continue, that people you had breakfast with will still be alive at suppertime. You have to trust that it is safe to have misunderstandings, separations, days off and off-days, time alone. You would go crazy if you had to live every second of your life as if it were the last.

But that is why death is such a shock: because you *cannot* be prepared for it and live a satisfactory life at the same time. Everyone is taken by surprise by a death: the trust that life *will* continue beyond lunchtime is always shattered when someone you love dies. *Everyone* is prone to reexamining the past in the light of this new, untrusting 'if only I'd known' perspective. The most important thing you can do, however, is accept that you could *not* have known; that you are not to blame for being human.

4

MOURNING TIME

The first year

It is impossible to think that I shall never sit with you again and hear your laugh. That every day for the rest of my life you will be away.

Dora Carrington

The prospect of the rest of your life stretching ahead without your parent can be extremely daunting. You may wonder how on earth you can survive these days, months and years to come. One day you think you are coping well, the next you feel worse than ever. Sometimes you can feel, as Dora Carrington did after the death of her beloved Lytton Strachey, that 'every day it gets *harder* to bear'.

If life is a journey, then grief is one of the roads we all, sooner or later, will travel along on the way. But grief is less like a smooth wide motorway than a potted, windy, bumpy, dirt track with very few lights and no signposts. Very often you end up wondering in despair if you are on the right road, having lost all sense of direction and distance, with no idea how far you are from your point of departure or your destination. At times it can be very hard to believe you are getting anywhere at all, and in the time ahead there may be moments of real desperation. Knowing this won't prevent these times of despair and disorientation, but the daunting prospect of a lifetime ahead without your parent can be made a little more manageable if you can anticipate some of the things that are likely to happen.

There is no foolproof timetable for mourning because everyone's reactions will be different according to their particular circumstances. But it is generally agreed that there a number of thoughts and feelings which most people tend to experience during the first few years after a bereavement. This is particularly true in the first two years. Knowing what these are can be a tremendous help, especially in those moments when you doubt you are making any progress at all.

It takes time

Coming to terms with a parent's death takes time. A lot of time. Without any serious disruptions or complications or further big losses during the first two years after a parent's death, you can still expect marked peaks and troughs in your emotions. Major events in the family, such as Christmas and birthdays, will be particularly difficult at first. By this I mean the *first few times* each one of these occasions is gone through, and apart from these times you can expect to go through 'lows' throughout the first two years, when you may feel unexpectedly overwhelmed with sadness or despair, anger or guilt, regret or resentment. Sudden floods of tears, or a spate of bad dreams and nightmares, colds and coughs, or just feeling lethargic or restless, are not unusual. All of these are a natural and normal part of adjusting to the major change that has taken place in your life.

I wish someone had explained to me about time when my father died. I wish someone had thought to tell me that a month is not long enough to get used to the death of someone who had been central to my life for eighteen years. It would have helped so much to know that however normal I might *appear* after a month, a year would not be long enough to begin to feel normal again. I so often caught myself saying crossly: 'Come on, girl. Pull yourself together. It's a long time ago now. You can't still be feeling miserable.' But I was. Sometimes I would be cross, sometimes impatient, sometimes sorry for myself, sometimes worried that I was *never* going to feel any better. Very rarely did it occur to me that actually 'it' wasn't very long ago at all. To lose someone you have lived with, loved with, fought with, eaten with, snuggled with for years and years, all your life in fact, whose presence is central to your experience of yourself takes far longer than the week between the death and the funeral.

It is thirty years since my father died. Sometimes that seems a long time ago, but occasionally, even now, it seems a recent occurrence, still fresh in my memory, still quick to pull at the heart strings. Even now, if I am under a great deal of emotional stress in my life, I can find myself pulled back to feelings I experienced in the immediate aftermath of my father's death. You do not ever entirely 'get over' the death of a parent, and you can ignore anyone who tells you so. To put it bluntly, they don't know what they're talking about. A parent's death is not a fence to be climbed over, or a stile to be crossed. It is an event which shapes your life from this moment on, just as, when still alive, your parent played a huge part in shaping your life. A parent's death profoundly alters your perspective on life. It changes the way you view friends and relatives; it can change your attitude towards life itself. You are not the same person after someone you love and need and care about has died, and to think of 'getting over it' is a waste of time. The very best you can hope to do – and in fact it *is* the very best you can do – is to adapt, be flexible, find ways of fitting into your changed world. You do not *get over* a death, but you can *come to terms* with it. It may not feel this way at first, but eventually you can learn how to fit death into life: how to find a place in your life for the experience that you have been through – and continue to go through.

The most helpful piece of advice I was given when my father died was by a friend of the family whose own father had died when he was a teenager. 'Don't expect to get over this,' he said. 'You won't. You don't ever get over it. You just get used to it.' It was good advice. Not waiting for a magical day when full recovery would arrive was very important. The idea of recovery is in many ways unhelpful; it implies that a major bereavement is similar to an illness. Instead of thinking in terms of 'getting over' your parent's death, thinking about 'getting used' to their death is a far more realistic and reachable goal. When a friend's mother died a year after my father, I passed on this advice. Later she wrote to me and said how helpful she too had found it. After all, imagine that every day for twenty years you have walked along a certain road and posted a letter at a certain letterbox. Then one day you walk along that road with your letter and find the box has gone. How long would it take to get over the absence of a mere letterbox? How much more important to you is a parent than a letterbox? The task of grieving is not to amputate your dead parent from your life, or to erase them from your mind and heart. The task of grieving is to move, gradually and at your own pace, towards making a new connection with your parent. Your mother or father is dead, but they are still part of your life, of who you are.

Talking cures

The second thing I wish I'd known was that allowing yourself to think and talk about the parent who died and your feelings about their death is not weak or self-indulgent or unhealthily morbid, but a vitally important means of adjusting to their absence. As Shakespeare put it in *Macbeth:*

> Give sorrow words; the grief that does not speak,
> Whispers the o'er fraught heart, and bids it break.

Talking is a way of remembering your parent that costs nothing but the energy, and perhaps the courage, it takes to remember. Through talking, or if talking is not possible at least allowing yourself to think about the parent you've lost, you help yourself to process the complex welter of feelings that are a normal part of mourning, and you begin the equally important task of finding a new way to stay connected to your dead parent. Numerous studies have shown that children who feel able to talk and think about their dead parent in the first year after the death are coping better and having fewer emotional problems after two years than those who have been discouraged from doing so. By talking, or thinking, about the things your parent said or did that mattered to you, that made you happy, that hurt you, that inspired you, that annoyed you, that delighted you, you honour the part they played in your life while they were alive and allow them to continue to have a place in your life even though they are now dead.

Talking and thinking about your parent are integral to the all-important process of building a new kind of relationship with your parent now that she or he is dead. Memories need not only be the positive things – remembering how your mother's disapproval used to cut you to the quick, or how your father complained about your table manners, can be as necessary as remembering things you loved about them. Remembering good things and bad, talking about them with friends and relatives, laughing together about the things you enjoyed and loved in the person who died, as well as the things that drove you crazy or hurt you, is an essential part of grieving and adjusting to what and who you have lost that was – and is – so important to you. The person who died not only caused pain and chaos by dying, he or she almost certainly also gave much of value and happiness to your life. It is worth remembering that. It is worth being proud of that memory and keeping it alive.

Whether or not it will be easy or even possible to talk varies hugely from one person to another. It will depend on your age, your personality, your gender, the relationship you have with your remaining parent, your family, your community, your culture, your religion, your everyday circumstances, your inner beliefs and attitudes. In some cultures talking about people who have died is acceptable and even expected. In others, it is considered morbid and unhealthy to talk about people who have died. Many traditional cultures think children should be kept away from anything to do with death, and adults actively discourage or prohibit children from talking about the dead. Even in cultures that allow adults to grieve and talk about dead loved ones, it is often felt by those same adults that death and youth are somehow incompatible. The truth could not be more different. Children are exposed to death at all ages and in all cultures all over the world. In the UK a child under 16 is bereaved every thirty minutes. One in twenty-five school-aged children today has experienced the death of a parent or sibling, and as many as 92 per cent of young people in the UK will experience a significant bereavement before the age of 16.[1]

MOURNING TIME: THE FIRST YEAR

The real reason that children are discouraged from talking about loved ones who have died, I believe, is that it makes the adults around them feel uncomfortable and out of their depth. Some years ago I was asked to give a talk about bereavement in a girls' secondary school. The proposed talk encountered a good deal of resistance from one of the teachers. Why did we need a talk on bereavement, she wanted to know. What was the point of upsetting everyone? It turned out this woman's mother had died when she was a teenager. It was not the pupils' feelings, but her own feelings that she didn't want to risk stirring up.

Children of all ages are very aware of the feelings of the people around them, and sensitive to their remaining parent's needs and emotions. Older children will often go to great lengths to conceal their feelings if they think that is what other people want them to do. They may take expressions such as 'you'll be the death of me' literally and believe that they are in some sense responsible for their parent having died. Fearing the apparently deadly power of their behaviour, they may then become overly obedient, compliant and good. Adults are all too likely to take this 'good' behaviour at face value, pleased that the child seems to be coping so well, relieved that there are no problems and failing to see that the good behaviour is just the public face of the child's anxiety and confusion. Adults in fact are not very good at recognising their children's distress and invariably underestimate their unhappiness.[2] When I asked a recently widowed father how his children were getting on, he replied in all seriousness, 'They seem to be fine.' His wife had died after a very short illness only eight weeks earlier. There was no way on earth his children were fine. Allowing himself to recognize their unhappiness was simply more than he could bear at that point in time, given the weight of his own grief, but my heart went out to his children all the same.

Janie was 9 years old when her mother died of cancer. She'd been vaguely aware of her mother's illness, but without understanding that her mother was going to die. No one had discussed the situation with her in any detail beforehand and her mother's death came as a tremendous shock. Janie wanted her father to comfort her, but also didn't like seeing her father upset. She tried hard not to show him, or anyone else, how upset and frightened she was feeling. She felt increasingly confused about what she was allowed to say and do, and as a result became quiet and withdrawn. Her father assumed this was a sign that she was coping well, and didn't realize how desperately she needed him to console and comfort her.

Children of all ages can feel silenced by a grief-stricken parent as well as by other relatives or family friends who seem to want them *not* to show their feelings. An Australian survey of 255 bereaved children under the age of 18 found that nearly all of them felt emotionally alone after their parent's death.[3] Very few had an adult they could talk to or discuss their worries with. One 13-year-old boy became very withdrawn after his mother's death. His father entirely misinterpreted his son's behaviour and took it as simple lack of grief. He told the interviewer his son was

> an odd, shallow little boy – he was very close to his mother and yet he never cried or said anything about her. He spends a lot of time in his room alone listening to records and doesn't help out around the house.

It seems hard to believe a father could so misinterpret his child's behaviour, yet it is far from uncommon. Even when remaining parents are very understanding and concerned, they are often immersed in their own grief, with little time or energy to spare for their children's needs in the first few weeks and months. Quick to pick up on the fragility of the surviving parent, as well as the new uncertainty hanging over the future, older children often try to conceal signs of their own distress. In the Australian study, for example, the most frequent reaction of 7- to 11-year-olds after a parent's death was to become silent or withdrawn. Other studies suggest that about half of all bereaved children will develop temporary problems of one kind or another in the first year after a parent's death.[4] When the father is the remaining parent, not talking and concealing emotions is more likely to be a problem, partly because fathers may be less inclined to talk to their children about their feelings and less skilled at doing so, partly because mothers are more likely to be very central to their children's daily lives, practically and emotionally, so their death hits children harder, and partly because they are simply overwhelmed by the task of taking over the running of domestic life, which is still generally done by mothers.[5]

While many children will go to considerable lengths to mask their feelings, others will try to express their distress and confusion indirectly by getting into trouble, being rebellious and aggressive, especially older children and teenagers. This kind of behaviour can happen at home, or more usually at school, where getting into fights or doing badly with school work can be a way of indirectly trying to get attention and support.[6] This kind of disturbance can start soon after the parent has died or may not appear for a year or more. It can last for a few weeks or for the rest of that child's time at school. What is nothing short of tragic is that teachers may be completely unaware that the child is bereaved and as a result rarely as supportive or sensitive to their needs as they could be. The compassionate intervention of a teacher at this stage can make a crucial difference in how a bereaved child adjusts to his or her loss, yet it is an intervention that even informed and caring teachers often fight shy of, embarrassed about broaching the topic of death, anxious about the kind of reception they may get, wary of upsetting the child. A number of teachers have expressed their belief to me that a bereaved child will most benefit from the normality of the school routine, and that the best approach is 'business as usual'. While there is certainly an element of truth in this, school children themselves experience considerable anxiety about the need to behave 'as if nothing had happened', often feeling that there is nowhere for them to express their feelings of dislocation and distress. Support programmes designed to give children space to talk about their feelings, if and when they want to, have been shown to help reduce this anxiety and sense of isolation.[7] At the very least, it helps children to know that what they are going through, however unpleasant it may be, is also normal and won't last forever.

The problem of finding space to grieve is particularly acute for children at boarding school. Twenty years ago, it was common practice to send children away when a marriage broke down or a parent died, either to school or to stay with relations, as if the child's feelings would diminish with distance. At boarding schools across the country today too there are grieving children who are assumed by the adults in their lives to be fine simply because they are a long way from home. A recent study of bereaved stepchildren disclosed heart-rending accounts of children as young as 5 sent to boarding school immediately after a parent's death, and given no opportunity or encouragement to come to terms with their loss. One girl even had a doll with clothes made for her by her dead mother taken away on arrival. Another was made to change the name on her schoolbooks to that of her stepfather. Even when a parent's desire – or a teacher's – to minimize a child's distress is entirely well-intended, the assumption that 'out of sight' is 'out of mind' is pure wishful thinking on the part of the adult, and in virtually every case only compounds the suffering of the grieving child.

In the past ten years, numerous studies have found that one of the big differences between young people who grieve for a dead parent without complications and those who have difficulty in grieving is whether or not they feel they have someone they can talk to about what they're going through.

The Child Bereavement Study in Boston found that children need various different kinds of communication after a parent's death.[8] First, they need clear and comprehensible information at the time of death and after in order to minimize their anxiety and fear of further abandonment and loss. They need to have their anxieties about the future heard and taken seriously, to have their needs for security, stability and safety taken into account. Younger children in particular need to know they are not to blame in any way for their parent's death. Second, children of all ages need someone to hear out their fears, fantasies and questions and not to have their feelings dismissed or discounted. Listeners do not need to be parents. They can be friends, teachers, counselors or other relatives. Third, they need reassurance that emotions, such as sadness, anxiety, guilt and anger, are a normal part of mourning, and to be given permission by adults around them to grieve in the way they want and to take the time to grieve that they need. When thoughts and feelings are especially over-whelming or intense, children and young people may need additional help and support to express these feelings in safe ways. Finally, they need opportunities to remember their parent, not just after death, but continuously throughout their life.

When I think back on my life in the year after my father's death, I can see that I had almost no one to talk to, either in my family or outside of it. I'd just left home to go to university. I was making new friends, but none of them knew me, or my father, or my family. I didn't want to talk to them about him anyway. Who'd want to be friends with someone who talked about a dead father the whole time? Besides, none of them had any idea what it was like to be bereaved. Or if they did, they were keeping as quiet about it as I was. Back home in the holidays, my mother was at full stretch, holding down a job, running the household single-handed, keeping going for my little brother and sister. She'd divorced my father many years before. There was not much overlap between my feelings about his death and hers. Looking back at my 18-year-old self, I can see how desperately lonely and isolated I was; at the time I just thought it was normal not to talk about 'it'. I didn't understand how much easier grieving for my father would have been if I'd had someone to turn to for support.

Families, like the individuals within them, differ widely in their incli-nation and ability to talk about difficult, sensitive subjects. Programmes and organizations that work with bereaved families can help parents and children to feel more comfortable with talking about the parent who has died and children's feelings and thoughts afterwards, but such help is not always available or affordable. A study of men whose fathers died when they were teenagers found that talking was not on the agenda in these households, for a range of different reasons, and this compounded the difficulties these sons were having in the aftermath of their fathers' deaths. The pervasion of the British stiff upper lip mentality meant that none of these boys had much opportunity to express or to process their grief within their families.[9]

If your family is religious, this too will affect how easily you are able to talk about your parent and your feelings about their death. Judaism is a religion that has a lot to recommend it in this respect, having developed a whole series of customs that make it easier for the bereaved to acknowledge their loss without embarrassment. Jewish funerals take place as soon as possible after the death, and immediately after the funeral a religiously observant Jewish family will sit *shivah* for seven days. During these official days of mourning they remain at home, receiving visitors and saying prayers. As Rabbi Jonathan Romain says in his book *Faith and Practice: A Guide to Reform Judaism Today*:

> The purpose of *shivah* is to be a comfort and help to the mourners. For centuries it has succeeded in being so, and has provided a structure both for the mourners to express their grief and come to terms with their loss, and for the surrounding community to give practical and emotional support.

After the seven days of mourning come the thirty days of *sheloshim* in which mourners begin to return to their normal lives, but traditionally do not go to parties or the cinema or theatre. After that comes the rest of the first year during which the bereaved are still recognized as being vulnerable and needing to grieve. To support people during this stage, special prayers are said at the weekly service. The end of the first year of life without the dead one is marked by the *Jahrzeit* or 'time of year' when the mourner lights a memorial candle in the home and says a prayer in synagogue. As well as lighting a yahrzeit candle and naming the deceased person's name in synagogue on the first anniversary of a death, Jewish people can do so *every single year* for as long as they wish to. Indeed, each week there is a part of the service given to saying 'kaddish', a prayer for the dead, in which anyone of any age can take a moment to remember people they have lost. Besides observing the anniversary of the person's death privately at home and publicly in synagogue, it is also acceptable and appropriate in Judaism to visit the cemetery at regular intervals, particularly on special occasions such as high holy days, a wedding anniversary, or the dead person's birthday. As Rabbi Romain explains: 'The Jewish way of mourning is a series of stages, each of decreasing intensity, which accompany the mourners from the first moments of grief and gradually return them to the stream of everyday life.'

I describe the Jewish mourning customs in detail because Judaism is one of the most helpful religions as far as coping with the day-to-day reality of bereavement is concerned. There is a lot of support from the community, and while excessive grief is not encouraged, the needs and feelings of mourners are respected and allowed, formally and informally, through specific traditions and customs and rituals, as well as through the attitude and sympathy of the community. The Jewish way of mourning allows people to grieve without shame. It makes grief acceptable and acknowledges that grieving is an important part of coming to terms with the death of someone you love. Most importantly, it acknowledges that dead people do not go away, but remain an integral part of your life. Even if you are not in the least religious, there is much in the traditional Jewish way of mourning that can be adapted to any bereavement.

'Two years is not too long'

The third thing to know is that two full years is not a long time when it comes to mourning for a parent's death.

In *Grief Counselling and Grief Therapy*, William Worden writes: 'Asking when mourning is finished is a little like asking how high is up? There is no ready answer. I would be suspicious of any full resolution that takes under a year, and, for many, two years is not too long.'

Worden wrote this in 1983 in a textbook for professional counsellors working with the bereaved. I picked it up in a bookshop one day, badly needing some information, from whatever source, about what was happening to me. Worden's cautious, measured phrase, 'For many, two years is not too long', was like a light coming back on in my head. So it was OK to feel this way twelve months after my Dad's death! It was not self-indulgent. I was not cracking up. In fact I had another twelve months to go! I was normal! Since then, much research into the experiences of bereaved children and teenagers has shown that the pattern of grieving is not quite the same in younger people as it is in adults. Worden's own research has found that symptoms of grief and problems associated with the death of a parent often only begin to emerge in children and teenagers during and after the second year following the death. In other words, two years may be just about when children and teenagers really *start* to grieve. In my work with bereaved school children, I have frequently found this to be the case. It can take up to a year or longer before the impact of a parent's death really begins to show. One problem that many young people face is that, by then, the adults around them will often fail to make the connection between their behaviour and the death of their parent. In teenage girls, for example, anxiety and problems linked to anxiety, such as difficulty concentrating on school work, are often worse a year or two after their parent's death, by which time, teachers and relatives may be slow to recognize the true cause of the apparent problem.

The funeral profession has got so skilful and quick at its job that it is easy to forget that the time taken to complete the necessary physical task – disposing of a body – has little bearing on the time it takes to get used to being without a fundamental part of your life, on how long we need to grow accustomed to these drastic changes in ourselves. Grieving for a parent is not an illness. It is a normal and healthy process of adjustment to a major life event, but not unlike a period of convalescence after a major illness, it is a period of time during which you may feel weaker than usual, more vulnerable to upsets, and more prone to feelings of sadness, despondency, and hopelessness.

It used to be thought that there were distinct stages to mourning. In her classic book on bereavement, *On Death and Dying*, published in 1970, Elizabeth Kubler Ross outlined five stages to grieving:

1st stage: Denial and isolation
2nd stage: Anger
3rd stage: Bargaining
4th stage: Depression
5th stage: Acceptance

The psychiatrist Colin Murray Parkes, in his book *Bereavement*, from the same decade, talks about four phases of mourning:

1st phase: Numbness
2nd phase: Yearning
3rd phase: Disorganization and despair
4th phase: Reorganization

For many years these 'phases' and 'stages' underpinned how grieving was viewed, and formed the basis for deciding if someone was grieving 'properly' or not. The drawback of viewing grieving in these ways is that it led for a long time to the idea that bereaved people should eventually reach a point in time when they are ready to 'give up' the dead person, to cast them off into the past and step out into one's own future. This idea has never made much sense to me. I have never understood why one is expected to amputate a dead parent from one's heart and mind like a rotten branch on an otherwise healthy tree. My dead father is as much a part of my self as my very alive mother. This was the case a week after he died, and a year after he died, and six years after he died, and it is still the case thirty years later. I have not only never reached a magical stage of 'letting go', but I have also stopped feeling vaguely anxious and guilty about my inability to 'let go'. I simply no longer see it as the desired goal.

Fortunately, in recent years, theories about grieving have caught up with what many of us always knew in our hearts. Phyllis Silverman, Director of the Child Bereavement Study at Massachusetts General Hospital, has presided over an important sea-change in the thinking about bereavement. She argues that the key task facing the bereaved is 'learning to remember', not learning to forget, and that 'coping [does] not involve recovery or resolution but [is] a process of adaptation and change'.[10] It has also been argued that the emphasis on letting go of the dead is culturally and temporally specific; in other words, other peoples in other places don't necessarily place the same importance as we in Britain and America tend to on forgetting people who have died, and, what is more, neither did we ourselves until this century. A study of twenty college women whose fathers had died revealed that 70 per cent still felt emotionally connected to their dead parent, and the large majority of those felt comfortable with that.[11] This finding has been replicated for other age groups. Instead of grief being seen as an inconvenient chore that has to take place in the first couple of years after someone you love has died, grieving is increasingly being regarded as a stage in a life-long process of adaptation. An American study in the 1980s found that even ten years after the loss, otherwise healthy people still experienced prolonged feelings of sadness, missing, crying, dreaming, so these kinds of feelings are not inherently abnormal.[12] Your relationship with your dead parent does not come to an end; instead, it continues to develop and change as you do, throughout your life. After a parent has died, the bond you have is no more static or fixed than it was when your parent was alive. Of course, people can get stuck in their relationship with a dead parent just as easily as with a living one, but it is the stuckness that is the problem, not the fact that there is a relationship.

Current approaches to mourning focus on tasks rather than on stages and phases. In *Children and Grief* William Worden outlines the following four main tasks:

Task I: To accept the reality of loss

A sense of disbelief after a death is normal. Disbelief can range from a hope that the loss has not really occurred to the full-scale delusion that the person is not dead at all. Over time, teenagers and adults realize and accept the reality that a loved one is dead and not coming back. Children also go through disbelief and a desire to deny the reality of death, and younger children may have particular difficulty with this, holding onto a belief that their parent is just 'away'. To accept the reality of loss is an essential task of mourning whatever your age, and it takes time.

Task II: To experience the pain or emotional aspects of the loss

Adults, children and young people all experience the same basic emotions after a major loss, but children and young people do not necessarily experience them in the same way as adults. Depending on their age, young bereaved people need to approach this task gradually and in ways that do not overwhelm them. A young person's ability to experience and process the pain of loss is highly influenced by how the adults around them are coping. If your surviving parent or carer can express grief openly and honestly without being overwhelmed, this sets a role model for positive mourning. You learn, by their example, that it is OK to feel terribly sad, to cry, to miss the dead person, and that these feelings although painful are survivable. Conversely, if the key adults in your life strenuously avoid showing any grief, or are overwhelmed or frozen by grief, you may become frightened of feelings in general and of your own feelings in particular. For young people, unused to and unprepared for the intense feelings of pain that accompany a major loss, this second task of mourning can be very difficult and may even be impossible until a long time, perhaps many years, after the actual death.

Task III: To adjust to an environment in which the deceased is missing

Adapting to the loss and change of roles within the family is an essential part of mourning, and will differ depending on an individual's personal circumstances, age and gender. In addition, the process of adjustment to how things have changed will itself change as a child grows older because the loss of a parent takes on new meanings and significance with time. What it means to be fatherless is not the same when you are 9 as when you're 19 or 39. This process of adaptation is a life-long process, not a one-off hurdle, because what your loss means to you continues to change throughout your life.

Task IV: To relocate the dead person within one's life and find ways to memorialize the person

This task too is ongoing and changing. It involves developing a new relationship with the person who has died, and making space to remember them in meaningful ways. This task is not accomplished once, but is very much a gradual, life-long process, one that will change as your feelings about your dead parent change over time, and as your needs and perspective change with age and subsequent events in your life.

No 'timetable' for grief can be anything but a rough guideline, because there is no way of determining exactly what you will feel and when. There is a wide variation in how people mourn. It depends on all sorts of factors that will be unique to your situation, your life, your personality, your past and future experiences as well as your present circumstances. No one can determine exactly how long your mourning will last because each of us is different. For some people, emotions will chase each other in a hectic circle; for others, one emotion will merge into another as time passes; other people may have very little feeling at all for a while, and then suddenly experience a great surge of grief.

What is helpful is to have some idea of the array of feelings which may possibly crop up at some point or other and in some form or other. Then at least you can look out for them and recognize them for what they are: normal reactions to loss, and normal ways of adjusting to the massive change that has taken place in your life. If you know what these feelings are and why you are feeling them, you can be less afraid of them, more patient with yourself, more able to tolerate the difficult and inevitably painful business of grieving.

Bad dreams and sleeplessness

You may well have vivid and often disturbing dreams in the first year after your parent's death. Dreams about your parent or about death generally are a feature of grieving by no means restricted to the first days, or even the first weeks after a parent dies. Dreams about your parent can continue all your life. But in the first year after the death, these dreams are common.

Carol's father had been very ill for almost a year and had recently gone into hospital. The afternoon that he died, Carol was in her flat in London, hundreds of miles away. She had been asleep after a hard week, and in her sleep she dreamt that her father came into the room, put his arm around her and, kissing her, said 'I'm all right. You don't have to worry about me. I'm fine. I just came to say goodbye.' Carol woke up very startled and immediately rang her mother. Her mother, however, said nothing was wrong, but she would ring if anything happened. Within five minutes her mother had called back to say she had been contacted by the hospital and Carol's father had in fact just died. In the weeks after his death Carol felt very comforted by the dream. 'I don't know whether it was real or not,' she says, 'but it was real to me and I felt he was telling me that he was all right. The funeral was a difficult occasion, people behaved pretty badly. It was really awful, in fact, but that dream really helped.'

Sometimes 'farewell' dreams can come a long time after your parent's death. Michelle was 16 when her father died. Almost a whole year later she dreamed that he came and sat on her bed, gave her a hug and said to her, 'You've got to let go of me now. It's time to let go of me and get on with your own life.'

But dreams are not always comforting personal farewells. Jeremy was there when his father collapsed and died of a heart attack and saw in detail what this entailed. For a year after his father's death, Jeremy had terrible nightmares, waking night after night in a cold sweat, terrified to go back to sleep again. Gradually his dreams became less frequent and less distressing, but while it was going on these months of interrupted sleep were very disturbing.

Sometimes dreams are comforting, sometimes they are not, but since there are so few other ways of going over the event of a parent's death, let alone one's feelings about it, dreams are our brain's natural way of doing so.

The week after her father died suddenly, Kate, who was 16 at the time, had a nightmarish dream that continued to trouble her on and off for many years. In the dream, she is in a car with her father, sitting in the back seat and looking out of the window as they drive along. Suddenly she realizes that they are about to crash and knows for certain they will both be killed. She tries to call out, to scream some warning to her father, but finds she cannot speak or move. She always wakes at the same moment: just as the car crashes. Kate sometimes still has this dream, although it is not always exactly the same. Her dream now often includes other people she cares about who are still alive. Sometimes she is in the car, sometimes she is watching from the pavement; always the people in the car are close friends or relatives. 'It's as if as soon as I care about anyone, I become convinced they are going to die,' Kate says. 'The worst thing about this dream, though, is that I can't do anything to stop them being killed.'

Kate's dream is disturbing but it is also a clue to unresolved feelings about her father's death, expressing her anxiety about being helpless and vulnerable in the face of death, unable to protect those she loves. It expresses her horror and shock that she could not prevent her father's death, as well as her continuing fears that such a thing could happen again. In this way, although it is painful and distressing, her dream is also trying to help her, by drawing attention to an area of emotional pain that she still needs to address in her waking life.

I continued to dream about both my father and my stepfather for years after their deaths, and still do occasionally. This is perhaps one of the clearest indications to me that it is totally unnatural to try to 'forget'. You simply do not forget someone who has been a key part of your existence. A parent remains in your memories and your thoughts whether or not you are always conscious of it. It takes a long, long time to come to terms with the death of someone who has meant so much to you, maybe a year or two actively, maybe ten years slowly and quietly beneath the surface. Dreams show just how gradual this process of accepting and understanding is; like continental drift, this process takes place invisibly, imperceptibly, inevitably.

Dreams are an ancient and vital part of the healing process. They are the mind's way of thrashing out fears and anxieties that might be too much to deal with directly at first. If possible try not to resist dreams, let them happen as and when they will, and maybe note down what happened in the dream when you wake up. Often the events of a dream seem bizarre the next day, but a week or a month later it will be easier to see what they 'mean'.

It is natural to go over and over an event which has affected you greatly. Think how the winning goal in a football match is relived time and time again, not only in action replays and sports highlights, but in conversation and imagination after the match. That night you lie in bed recalling the line of the ball as it sailed into the net, hearing again the roar of the crowd, feeling the surge of exhilaration in your chest. Or think how you felt after making a public speech, or acting, or playing in a concert. If it goes well you want to relive the moment, and if it goes badly you can't help reliving it! Think of the cliché of the mother who goes on and on about what her daughter's first child has learnt to do. Think how after a party you can't wait to phone friends or see them the next day to discuss every single aspect of it all over again.

Moments of significance in one's life call to be repeated in thoughts and words long after the event. When the events are happy or triumphant ones, this is accepted as perfectly normal: *you* might not want to watch the video of Christine and James' wedding for the tenth time, but you can understand that they do. When the events are difficult, painful, frightening and tragic, however, we try to put them out of our mind. Yet the need to relive the moment is as great, if not greater, in tragic or traumatic circumstances. It is how you make sense of the extraordinary, how you give the momentous a place in your everyday life. People *need to* do this, both in joyful and in tragic situations.

Studies of children and teenagers interviewed for the Child Bereavement Study in America show that dreaming about one's dead parent is not only a normal part of grieving, but also a healthy part of grieving: 50 per cent of Child Bereavement Study children dreamed about their dead parent during the first four months after the death, and 54 per cent *still* dreamed about their parent after two years.[13] Interestingly, the children who had dreamed about their parent four months after the death were finding life easier after two years than those who had not dreamed about their parent in the weeks and months immediately following their death.[14] Often, *not* dreaming is more of a cause for concern, a sign that the necessary process of adjustment is not yet happening. One girl, who had not dreamt about her father since his death when she was 13, only began dreaming about him after a year had passed. Dreaming made her sad, but at the same time the feeling of having 'found' her father again was very comforting. A man of 40 whose mother died when he was 17 told me that he has still never dreamed about his mother to this day. 'There is a gap deep inside me where she should be,' he says. 'I haven't felt ready to face that gap until now, but now I do. I'd always felt frightened of dreaming about my mother, but now I want to. I'm ready for her to be part of my life again.'

Dreams have an important, if sometimes painful, role to play. If you didn't see how your parent died, your imagination tries to supply the information. There are so many unanswered questions, horrible possibilities and frightening ideas, yet you can't ask anyone about these things for fear of seeming macabre or morbid, so you explore these possibilities in your sleep, through dreams. Dreams allow you to continue in your imagination the relationship that death had brought prematurely to an end. Dreams are a way of supplying answers to the now unspoken questions in your head. Persistent bad dreams can make you feel that sleep is your worst enemy, but if possible try to see dreams as 'useful' rather than good or bad. As the novelist William Golding, writing in the twentieth century, said:

> Sleep is when all the unsorted stuff comes flying out as from a dustbin upset in a high wind.

Dreams are giving you an opportunity to look at the 'unsorted stuff' and make some sense of it.

Sleeping pills, tranquillizers and antidepressants

Biologically sleep is necessary: deprived of sleep we eventually go crazy, and long before that we become irritable, cannot concentrate, feel nauseous and shaky. It is better to have some sleep than none at all. If you are really distressed by continually troubling dreams then it is worth going to see a counsellor, therapist or priest to work out precisely what is troubling you and how to cope with it. If you are becoming very sleep-deprived and finding it hard to cope during the day as a result, medication can be helpful but it should only be used as a temporary measure. Talk to your GP or pharmacist, as there are a number of herbal remedies that can help with sleep. Since sleeping pills, tranquillizers and antidepressants all effectively dull your distress, they can seem an attractive option, but they have been shown also to slow the process of absorbing what has happened. This can end up making matters worse, not better, in the long run. It is like entering a time capsule to avoid a war – you still step out to the same devastation. Attempting to dull your senses at this critical time may even make it harder to come to terms with what has happened by increasing the feeling of dislocation and unreality without alleviating the pain. Taking pain-killers before plunging your hand into boiling water might stop it hurting so much in the short term, but it doesn't do anything to help the burn. I was put on antidepressants by my GP eight months after my stepfather died and although I hated the sensation of being drowsy and inert, as if wrapped in a heavy blanket, nevertheless I did sleep through the night for the first time in months, and the silence in my head for a while was a relief. For someone in a thoroughly exhausted state, tranquillizers and sleeping pills may just help by allowing you to break the pattern of sleeplessness with a run of solid ten-hour nights. For some people pills can provide a necessary bridge between the intense agitation caused by a parent's death and a slightly calmer state in which you can begin to mourn more effectively. What they cannot do is release you from the need to grieve, nor eradicate the pain of loss.

The first six months

After the funeral everyone goes back to their normal lives and you are left to try and find some way of getting back to yours. These weeks can be very difficult. Sudden swings of emotion; enormous sadness; sleeplessness; confusion – all are feelings to be expected at this time. Support from close friends and relatives usually continues for a little while, but rarely for long enough. For the many people who no longer belong to traditional reli-gious communities, there is not much in the way of formal structures for supporting the bereaved. Most people tend to go back to school or uni-versity or work within a few days of the funeral, and this can provide important daily structure and diversion from thoughts and feelings of grief, and the yawning gap left by your parent's death. For many young people, in particular, the pressure of ordinary life can feel quite burdensome at this time, however. You may feel you have to pretend to be fine when you feel anything but. You may find it hard to concentrate, or feel your routine activities are pointless. Lack of sensitivity and support from those around you can make you feel more alone with your grief. These feelings are all normal and understandable, however painful.

Coping with the outside world

Whether you want it or dread it, the return to school, college or work can be very hard. Often it throws you into a situation where very few people know what has happened to you or make allowances for you. The pressure to cover your feelings, avoid embarrassing shows of emotion and appear as normal as possible is very strong. But very likely you will be feeling far from normal, often far *more* touched by death than before.

When I went back to college after my stepfather's death I felt as if I had some kind of disease and that other people could see it just from looking at me. I imagined they were afraid of being contaminated by this death that had so afflicted me. Surrounded by college friends, I felt incredibly lonely, shut inside a glass bubble, unable to reach the world and unable to be reached by it.

Other people's awkwardness and embarrassment can be very hurtful. Hugh was working as a young student teacher when his father died. He went back to work after the funeral and found it a most wounding experience. No one said anything at all about his father's death.

> There was only one other teacher who spoke to me and even he was too embarrassed to ask directly how I was, but he did ask how my mother was doing. He kept asking after her, even several months later. It was an indirect way of showing concern for me and I really appreciated it. It made a lot of difference.

At school you have to cope with other people's embarrassment; you have to cope with exams and homework; you have to put up with the dramas of friends, which in comparison to the death of a parent may seem pathetically trivial. Even your closest friends can run out of sympathy surprisingly quickly.

At work you try to appear normal when in fact you are feeling strange and unlike yourself. You have to rise to challenges that you may not feel up to yet. It is not unusual, after a major bereavement, to feel withdrawn, easily tired, lacking in energy and confidence, especially if you are distracted by worries about your family. If it is your first job and important to you to do well, this can be another source of pressure.

Adults who lose a parent can also find it hard to make sense of what has happened when the relentless demands of small children, the household chores and work commitments can leave very little space for grieving. The pressure to carry on as usual and get back to normal can be hard to resist. It can even feel quite welcome for a while, but if it becomes in the least stifling or oppressive, it is very important to allow yourself to have some 'time out'. Young children do this instinctively after a major bereavement – they will behave quite normally, playing games, laughing and chatting, and then will become agitated, angry, upset. It is as if they introduce themselves to their grief in small stages. Teenagers and adults find that much harder to do.

It can be hard to say to teachers or employers 'Give me a break. This is a hard time for me.' You feel you are making excuses and may be worried that they will think so too. Society demands from the young unflagging energy, drive, commitment, enthusiasm and confidence. It is not very tolerant of the effects of bereavement. You yourself may be the least tolerant of all.

David's mother died at the beginning of his final year of school. With A levels approaching, he felt under great pressure to keep working for his exams and not allow his feelings about his mother's death to overwhelm him. To begin with, he seemed to be managing to keep his emotions in check, but the Christmas holidays broke the rigid routine he had imposed upon himself, and the following term he found it increasingly difficult to concentrate on his school work, was frequently depressed, and began to have anxiety attacks. When a teacher suggested that David might benefit from being given an extension with his A level coursework, he rejected the idea, thinking that to agree would be a sign of weakness and failure on his part. He felt that he *ought* to be able to cope, and that applying for an extension would just be an excuse. He couldn't see the pressure he was under, nor how reasonable it was in the circumstances that he should *not* be coping.

A year or two after my father's death, I was interviewed for a job by the BBC. The interviewer kept badgering me to explain why I hadn't watched Breakfast TV when it first started. He thought it showed a lack of interest. I thought he should have read my C V more carefully. When he asked for the third time why I had nothing to say about breakfast television, I snapped back, 'Because it coincided with my father dying and I had other things to think about!' I didn't get the job, needless to say, but I was glad I'd spoken up.

Having your experience denied and being made to feel somehow invisible does not help you settle back into school or work. It hurts to be made to feel like a social pariah, the person no one wants to have around, the misery-guts, the harbinger of doom and gloom. When I went back to school after my father died I found it very upsetting that no one actually asked how I was, neither teachers nor pupils. No one mentioned that I had been off school for a week. Some people clearly avoided me, and if that was not possible, evaded any form of conversation that might bring up the dreaded topic of death.

In these situations, where others seem intent on avoiding all mention of what has happened, or perhaps genuinely do not know what has happened, it can be helpful to tell certain people who need to know, such as bosses, tutors, headteachers. It is important that they can take into account the fact that you are reeling from a parent's death when it comes to assessing your behaviour – as they have to do. If they do not know the circumstances, it is hard for them to understand why you cannot do your homework or are not meeting deadlines; that you are feeling miserable and your concentration is shot to pieces; that you can't sleep at night for bad dreams; that the rest of the family is in a similar state of disarray; that you may be moving from the home where you have lived all your life; that your mother is working longer hours to make up the shortfall in the family income; and that you now have to shop on the way home from school and make supper every night, and afterwards are simply too tired to do your homework. Not all teachers, tutors or employers will turn into sensitive, caring, tolerant people, but some might – and anything that helps you right now is worth a try. In the case of David, quoted earlier, he eventually did agree to apply for an extension for his A level coursework, the extension was readily given, and David experienced a tremendous sense of relief as a result.

This is a profoundly distressing period, when your feelings are somehow not your own, and there are very few guidelines or supports. How normal should you be? How happy is it OK to be? How *unhappy* is it OK to be? Can you talk about your father or mother? Should you be spending more time at home?

This is a time when you may well feel fine for a day or two, and then, just when you think you are 'over it', you crash, and find yourself feeling more wretched than you did before. Each time you think you're over the worst, another wave of sorrow engulfs you, more powerful than the last. In his account of his wife's death and its aftermath, *A Grief Observed*, C.S. Lewis describes these sudden pangs of grief:

> There comes a sudden jab of red-hot memory and all this 'commonsense' vanishes like an ant in the mouth of a furnace.

In these first months you can often feel torn between wanting life to resume as quickly as possible, wanting to stop thinking about death and pain and loss and, on the other hand, wanting to keep the dead person alive in some way – through talking about them, mentioning their name, thinking about them, wearing their clothes. These two desires – to remember and to forget – can exist at the same time.

Helen, whose mother died when she was 17, could not bear to be at home where everything was so gloomy and morbid, but every time she went out with her friends she felt guilty. She felt she ought not to be having a good time, felt guilty for trying to forget. She needed friends to make her feel more normal, but felt wrong for appearing to 'recover' so quickly after her mother's death.

I remember similar feelings: being completely fed up with being different from my friends, but somehow not really quite being able to enjoy the things they were doing. After one party the gap between the fun everyone else seemed to be having and the fun I was trying and failing to have was too much: I broke down in tears, to the bewilderment of friends, and just howled for about an hour. Everything looked so black. I didn't want to be bereaved, I wanted to be like everyone else. I wanted to forget about death and grief and pain, but it seemed impossible.

Fear of forgetting

You may find yourself afraid that you will forget your parent, as scared of getting better as you are of not getting better. I was torn between wanting to forget what had happened and being scared of forgetting. But this fear of forgetting is unfounded: there is no chance that you will forget. Despite your fears, the memory of a person is not like a photograph that fades with time. Your anxiety that you will lose the dead person utterly if you forget them for a moment is also baseless. There is no harm in trying to forget from time to time. It is not wrong to smile, laugh, have fun and enjoy yourself after someone has died. Constant unrelieved feelings of anxiety, fear and pain lead eventually to serious depression and ultimately to complete breakdown. You need to have moments off from grief – if only to recharge your batteries for coping with the next bout of sorrow. Often enough, it will not seem possible to find enjoyment in life, so when the opportunity arises to feel OK for a while, don't feel guilty about it, be grateful for it. It is not wrong, it is absolutely essential. You need these moments of respite. Even a screaming child is silent in the moments when it is drawing breath.

There are no rules. If the first week before the funeral is a phase of limbo-chaos, this is a phase of active-turmoil, a phase of mirrors and mirages, where nothing is as it seems, nothing feels solid or reliable. Stick with it and try to trust that you will eventually come out the other side into a more substantial world.

Six months to a year

You can still expect to feel considerable grief six months after a parent's death. Your moods will continue to be unpredictable. 'Red-hot memory' can still play havoc with your emotions, and you may well find that only now is the fact of your parent's death and its implications for the rest of your life beginning to sink in. Depression and anger about a parent's death are often slow to emerge and it is now, seven or eight months later, when you expect to be 'better', that you may instead feel particularly vulnerable and unhappy.

Emerging emotions

After my father's funeral was over I did not cry again for six months, and it was closer to eight months before I could really begin to look at his death straight on and face what it meant. Until then I was on hold, pretty miserable, just about coping, but not really getting anywhere in terms of making sense of his death and what it meant for me.

It took eight months for me to discover, as many others have, that depression is one aspect of mourning that tends to appear later rather than sooner. Just when I thought things were beginning to settle down, after the initial shock had worn off and the anger had subsided and the acute pain of missing my father had lessened, it was only *then* that I found myself struggling with thick, heavy, leaden despair.

This delayed reaction is in part a mechanism to protect you from the full impact of a death until you are ready to cope with it. You need a great deal of energy and emotional reserves simply to keep going in the first six months, and some things have to wait for a while.

My father's death coincided with my year off before going to university. A few months after he died, I set off as planned to work on a campsite in France. There was a lot to cope with: I had left home for the first time; I was without my friends, my family and my belongings for the first time; I was in a new place, doing a new job, living with new people. To begin with, I was simply too busy to have time to grieve. It wasn't until life settled down on the campsite that my feelings began to emerge. With the routine life, the quiet afternoons and the distance from people I knew and cared about, it became possible to think about what had happened – and to begin to feel it too. But it came as a shock to be feeling these things so long after the event. I thought I'd already done despair and loneliness and confusion. I thought it would be a gradual return to normality from month three onwards.

Grief, as I found out, has its own timing and is not averse to going back and doing certain things again. Grief is a maze which builds itself as it goes along, blocking off an entrance here, making an exit there, darting back on itself, advancing in mysterious, twisting routes which rarely feel like an advance to those stuck in it. Professionals may pick out clear patterns, but their perspective is different. For those in the maze, no pattern is usually visible.

Another emotion that was still causing me trouble at this time was anger. Eight months after my father's death, I wrote in my diary:

> I miss Dad so much. Not just as sadness, but as an enormous anger. I feel angry, angry, angry – that I shall never know him, nor he me. And I feel angry that I wasted the last years of his life with my friends, instead of with him. All the memories I have of Dad are spoiled with regret, bitterness, guilt. Even three more years and I might have come to know him a little. It makes me so sad and angry. I so want to know him, and I can't. It's just not fair. That's what I feel – like a spoilt child who can't have what she wants. I miss him so much and often I find myself on the verge of tears. If only, only, only there'd been time to know him a bit.

This feeling of having been cheated is common after someone dies, particularly a parent who has died when you are both still relatively young. I have heard plenty of people utter this complaint: that someone and something has been taken away unfairly, the rules of the game have been changed without any warning, the goalposts moved while your back was turned.

What has been taken away is not just a person you needed to be alive still, but also time. Time to do your own thing, time to get to know your parent as a person, time to fight and make up with your family, time to get away from them for long enough to get to know yourself a bit, time to be young and carefree, time to be selfish and independent. Anger, under the circumstances, is a normal emotion and one that many bereaved children feel. It is an emotion that needs to be given space and looked at with understanding and compassion for yourself.

Lack of support

You can feel very alone in the maze at this stage. Relations you had relied on in the early days to give support may well be withdrawing into themselves to try to cope with their own loss. Friends can find it hard to remember that seven or eight months, which seems a long time to them, is no time at all for you.

After her mother died, Maria had to leave home and move to Edinburgh to start her first year as an undergraduate. She was determined to cope, determined to keep up appearances of being just like all the other students. 'In the end,' she says, 'I made myself ill with the effort of pretending.' At the end of her first year she dropped out and came back to London. Her friends were little help:

> They couldn't understand what I was going through. And because I had had a difficult relationship with my mother and had often complained about her when she was alive, some of them even said to me, 'But you didn't like your mother, did you? Why are you so upset?' They really couldn't see. I used to feel very angry with them for not understanding. And of course they expected me to be over it in a week.

The only person whom Maria did feel at ease with was a girl she didn't know that well, but whose own mother had died not long before. They rarely spoke explicitly about what they were thinking and feeling, 'but I knew she basically understood what it was like. We just used to sit in silence a lot of the time, but it was better than being with other friends who expected me to be just like them.'

For children and teenagers in particular, lack of support is a common problem. One study found that around the time of the death and funeral, 42 per cent of children felt pressure to behave a certain way for surviving parent's sake.[15] Girls were more likely to talk to a surviving parent or friend about the death than were boys, and teenage boys in particular were likely to be told to be 'grown up' and keep their feelings under control and out of sight. Almost half of the children in this study had nobody they felt they could talk to about their dead parent, and 14 per cent felt at risk of teasing or bullying because of having a dead parent / only one parent. An 11-year-old broke down in tears as she told the interviewer how other children bullied her about not having a father. A 12-year-old was taunted by a neighbour's child: 'Ha, ha, you don't have a mother and I do.'[16]

The fact that friends have seldom been through a bereavement means they simply cannot know how long grief lasts, and inevitably this can leave you feeling very isolated and abandoned. You can also feel envious of other people for *not* knowing what you are going through, envious of the fact that they are not going through it themselves. Many of the children in the Childhood Bereavement Study told the interviewers how hard they found it when other children complained about their living parents. 'You're lucky you don't have a father,' a child with two parents told a 6-year-old boy whose father had died. A 16-year-old boy said: 'You hear kids, like, say they hate their parents and stuff. It's like you don't know how much you like them until you lose them.'[17]

Being with friends and their parents at cheerful family occasions sometimes felt comforting, but more often it can leave you feeling like an outsider, very lonely, and often envious. Sometimes friends will have complicated reasons of their own for failing to be as supportive as you need them to be. I remember admitting to a close friend in a moment of honesty, how wretched I was feeling, that I was struggling to cope with the deaths of my father and stepfather in such quick succession. I could not see a way forward, I confessed. She suddenly lost her temper and snapped back at me, 'For God's sake, pull yourself together. My father walked out on me and Mum when I was 4. You're not the only person in the world not to have a father. Stop making such a big deal of it.' I was astounded. How could she be so cruel? So incredibly unsympathetic?

Later on I was able to see that maybe she was right, that she had been bereaved in a way when her parents separated. To a 4-year-old that too would have felt like a dreadful loss. The sense of being unentitled to your feelings is as great when you lose a parent that way and at that age; certainly other people are more sympathetic when there is something clear and unambiguous like a death. I could see how her own feelings of loss might have been reactivated by my situation and her angry outburst came to seem more understandable.

Lack of sympathy and support from friends is usually due simply to ignorance. The problem of how to cope with bereavement at an age when so few of your contemporaries know what you are going through is a very real one. You are out of step with your peers and not much can be done to change that. Your needs are very different from theirs. You are highly sensitized to a whole dimension of life that to them is still theoretical, abstract, impersonal, an easy source of humour, not the painful reality that leaves you often in or close to tears.

I once disgraced myself – or so I felt – when I went to the cinema with a group of friends whom I hadn't known for long and didn't know very well. The film was very funny, until one of the characters, a man in his mid-forties, had a heart attack and died. While everyone else roared with laughter, I burst into tears. My father had had a heart attack in his late forties, and watching the man on the screen was just too near the bone. But I was ashamed of my outburst and it certainly put a damper on the evening. Others have had similar experiences: a few weeks after Jocelyn's mother died, a friend tried cheering her up by taking her to *Indiana Jones and the Temple of Doom*. She too burst into tears – all the intended 'funny' scenes which involved any violence, threat to life, or actual death, were just too distressing for her to cope with. *Once Upon a Time in the West* was so unfunny to a bereaved 21-year-old that he had to leave after the first ten minutes, much to his well-intentioned friend's dismay.

Children who do feel able to speak with friends about their bereavement seem to feel more connected to their dead parent, and they also have higher levels of self-esteem than those who do not.[18] Yet it is not at all uncommon not to have anyone you feel comfortable talking to, either your remaining parent or people of your own age. Teenage girls are most likely to talk to friends in the early days after a parent's death, followed by pre-teen girls. Boys of all ages are least likely to talk to friends about a dead parent, in particular pre-teen boys.[19]

The Childhood Bereavement Study found a range of reasons why it can be difficult or uncomfortable to talk to friends and why bereaved children often don't want to. These include:

- Fear of crying or getting emotional:

  'I don't want them making fun of me' – 10-year-old boy whose father died.

- The subject never comes up:

  'My friends think I should be over it. They don't say so. It's just the way they look at me' – teenage girl whose mother died when she was 11.

- Friends are trying to be protective:

  'They think if they keep talking about it, I'll get sad because in the past I've gotten sad talking about it. They just don't want me to get sad. I just want them to listen. I can't blame them because they never had their father die' – 11-year-old girl.

- Awkwardness on the part of friends:

  'They knew my father had died, but I don't think they knew how to act' – pre-teen girl.

- Not knowing:

  'Most of my friends don't know about my father' – 9-year-old girl two years after her father's death.

- Not caring:

  'I don't talk to friends about my mother. I guess they don't really care. They're interested more in sports than in listening to me' – 11-year-old boy.

- Circumstances of the death:

  'I've never told them that he died [by suicide] 'cause they would tell everyone else and then they will ask me about the death' – 6-year-old girl whose father killed himself.

- Feels too personal:

  'In school I don't want everybody knowing my business. I don't tell them nothing!' – 15-year-old girl.[20]

Relationships

Feeling out of step with your peer group puts a strain on relationships too. One common effect of a bereavement is to make you fearful of other people dying. Anxiety about a partner, being frightened by separations and absences are very understandable in the circumstances, but can nevertheless cause real problems when it comes to girlfriends and boyfriends. Partners often don't understand; they interpret it as clinginess, over-dependence and over-involvement, and may be scared off by the way they see this fearful reaction. They want to be having fun, not coping with your grief and anxiety. But fun is not particularly easy to have when your world is thrown upside down and turned inside out, when everything around feels dangerous, fragile and unreliable. What do you do? Do you pretend? Do you avoid any connection with other people, so that your needs and fears remain hidden?

There are no easy answers. The only solutions are short term: be kind to yourself, put your needs high up the scale of priorities, try not to deny your feelings in the hope of pleasing other people. Give yourself time to grieve: it won't go on forever, and it is far better to feel these things now than to store them up for later.

As far as navigating your way through the minefield of a relationship is concerned – a minefield for all people whatever their age or stage of life, bereaved or not – you can only really aim to be honest with yourself, to accept the way you are feeling, not to compromise too much, not to force yourself to pretend too often. Allow yourself to feel how you feel, and to be the way you need to be. This may not make you great company at times, but friends and partners worth having will understand and make allowances. At least this course of action will allow you to get on with grieving and coming to terms with grief, a process which is invariably hampered by hiding your feelings, ultimately with the greatest damage to yourself.

Coping with family conflict

Grief does not take place in a vacuum. It is located in a family's emotional culture. How you and your family react to a bereavement will depend not only on the immediate circumstances surrounding the death, but on how emotions and problems are handled in your family. If your parents always tried to present a united front to the children, seldom expressing or discussing personal thoughts and feelings, it will be more difficult for them to share their grief and more shocking and frightening for you if they do so. Equally important is your temperament: some people are naturally more expressive or more restrained than others, which is one reason why two siblings in the same family may react differently to a parent's death.

If you are still living at home when a parent dies, strife between you and other members of your family may be a problem. You may feel very out of step with other members of your family – either because they still seem stuck in a more intense state of grief than you, or because they seem to be coping much better than you. Or you may feel angry about how family life has changed since your parent's death. Conflict between teenagers and their remaining parent is common as everyone has to adjust to new routines, new ways of doing things, new rules and ways of dealing with differences.[21]

One 19-year-old was infuriated by her mother's refusal to throw out any of her dead father's clothes. She wanted to get them out of the house; only then would she really be able to get on with her life again. But her mother was not ready; it made her feel safe having her husband's clothes around, as if a bit of him were still with her. Her justification that it would somehow be disrespectful to get rid of the clothes 'so soon' exasperated and distressed her daughter, who found the sight of her dead father's suits hanging in the cupboard morbid, not comforting.

Different ways of expressing grief can cause conflict too: Hattie's mother and younger sister talked and cried openly, which she found hard to handle. Hattie, who was 13, wanted only to be left alone with her thoughts and feelings. She didn't want to join in these emotional displays which she found self-indulgent and embarrassing. She was irritated and revolted by what was for them very helpful.

Every member of a bereaved family has her or his own private feelings to deal with, and inevitably needs will be different. There is always room for tension in any family, and at a time such as this stress is not surprising. A common source of conflict – expressed or concealed – is the role of older siblings, relatives or family friends who have stepped in as a kind of surrogate parent; an intrusion you may deepy resent. The 'helpful' words and deeds of an aunt, uncle or friend of the family may seem to you interfering and wholly unwelcome. The unwanted presence may increase your feelings that your life has been disrupted and destroyed by death and that nothing will ever be good again. For you, it may make matters worse not better that a neighbour cooks supper for you all, or that an uncle now helps your mother with bills and accounts. For you, your parent is irreplaceable and these pseudo-parents only emphasize what you have lost. In no way do they begin to make up for it. When widowed parents are asked how their children are coping with the death of a parent, they often reflect instead on how they themselves are feeling. This is particularly true of domestic arrangements. If your widowed father has arranged for a family friend to be at home when you get back from school, he will probably be relieved to have solved that problem at least and assume his children are too. The truth may be very different. Your resentment, anger, irritability and hostility are not easy feelings to cope with, but neither are they entirely unreasonable in the circumstances: it is understandable that a person stepping into your dead parent's shoes should be more an irritating presence than a soothing one to you. They stand, literally, for what you have lost. It is natural not to welcome them with open arms, even if you can accept that they are helping in practical ways. The fact that they are there at all reminds you that others are not.

It is important in this situation to try to hold both realities in mind: the fact that you do not want a surrogate parent, and the fact that you and your family may really need the practical help that this person can give, be they brother, sister, uncle, aunt or neighbour. Allow yourself to appreciate their help and good intentions, but equally you can allow yourself your feelings of hostility and resentment: they are a valid part of your grief, an expression of the anger that you feel. After all your world has been overturned and undergone these profoundly unwanted changes. You need not act on these feelings, but neither do you need to deny their existence.

Relationship with the parent who has died

More difficult to handle are the after-effects of a complicated relationship with the parent who has died. Tony Walter makes the point that: 'It is not the quality but the *intensity* of the relationship with the deceased that is crucial, and the hardest grief can be for those close family members with whom you did not get on.'

Jane always argued with her mother, and after her mother's death Jane was left with dreadful feelings of guilt, imagining that she had made life difficult at home for everyone, and that she might somehow have caused her mother's cancer by being so quarrelsome. The phrase 'you'll be the death of me' suddenly sounded quite different to Jane's ears.

Sean, on the other hand, had a very cool relationship with his mother and was very close to his father. When his father died he was left feeling guilty that he had not been nicer to his mother who was now all he had. He also felt guilty for secretly wishing his mother had died and not his father.

Another cause for conflict at this time can come when there are stepparents or stepchildren in the family. A stepparent may well have brought you up from an early age and been a crucial figure in your life, but you may find after his or her death that your grief is somehow invalidated because you were not blood relatives. I know how hurt I was when in the obituary for my stepfather I read that he would be mourned by 'his widow and four children'. What about me and my brother? Did we not count? Had we not loved him too? Had we not been loved by him? Had he not taken us to school, bathed us, fed us, read us bedtime stories, picked us up when we fell, cuddled us when we cried? Was he not a father to us too? Were we not entitled then to mourn the man who had brought us up for the last fifteen years? Was our grief to be dismissed so easily? Nor were careless journalists the only ones to dismiss my sorrow and loss: friends and relatives also somehow seemed to assume that I felt less because he was 'only' my stepfather.

Yet as Tony Walter points out, often we grieve hardest for those whom we may have had difficulties loving, and between stepparents and stepchildren the bonds of affection are often extremely complicated – a maze of dependence, gratitude, love, anger, resentment, hostility: a whole hotch-potch of negative and positive emotions that can make the grief you feel when they die all the more difficult to cope with.

The fact that society can often fail to recognize the very powerful – though not straightforward – bonds between steprelatives can be an additional source of pain and anger at an already difficult time. Step-siblings can be regarded as more affected by the stepparent's death than you; you may feel your relationship with your stepparent is overlooked. This is incredibly painful and distressing, when it happens, and the first thing you must do in this situation is to tell yourself that whatever anyone else thinks, you are entitled to your grief too.

There is also the possibility that your blood-parent may have been the one to die, leaving you with a stepparent for whom you may have ambivalent feelings or with whom you have a strained relationship. Anne's mother died when she was 6. Her father remarried two years later, but he then died a year after that, leaving Anne and her three brothers in the care of their new stepmother. At the age of 65, Anne looks back with understanding and also regret at a situation that was extremely difficult for everyone.

> My stepmother was a good woman and she did her best, but we hardly knew her. It was impossible for her to replace both my parents. My brothers and I were close, but we never talked about our feelings. We all just had to get on with life as best we could.

In situations like these you may well have to cope with emotions and thoughts that seem unacceptable and shameful. Why didn't your stepparent die instead? Maybe you felt that he/she was responsible for the death in some way – maybe if the ambulance had been called sooner, or your parent had been made to lose weight, or stop smoking. All kinds of feelings of suspicion and hostility towards a stepparent that have been hidden away can come flooding to the surface in the aftermath of a parent's death. And if you are still dependent on your stepparent for a home, food, financial support and so on, the sensation of being both abandoned and trapped can be very distressing. After all, maybe you never even wanted this person in your life, and now you're somehow stuck with them for good. Even if you are financially independent, you may feel responsible for a stepparent after a parent's death. Wanted or not, the emotional ties to a stepparent can be strong. They now represent your links with the parent who has died; you may feel that you need them now in some way. If you break away from them, you will risk losing still more of your links with your dead parent. Whatever the relationship with your stepparent, there are nearly always conflicting and ambivalent feelings to cope with.

There are several organizations designed to help with the complex emotional ties within stepfamilies (see p. 213–5), and it may be worth your while contacting them for support. For the time being, it is important that you recognize and accept the validity and reality of what you are feeling. Give yourself permission to be angry, frightened, lonely, resentful. Give yourself permission to mourn the loss of a stepparent who mattered to you, and give yourself permission to have mixed feelings about a step-parent you are now left with. A bereavement may provide an opportunity to look honestly at emotions that have never before seen the light of day. Be honest with yourself. Accept your reaction to your parent's death, and give some room to all the conflicting, contradictory, negative emotions and thoughts that may, understandably, be troubling you.

5

MOURNING TIME

The second year and after

Death produces a sudden nothingness in the world, a hole in the
fabric of the world, with which the survivor must learn to live,
and whether the lost one be loved or hated makes no difference,
that learning still is difficult.

John Banville

When a parent dies it leaves a gap not only inside you, but also in the
world you live in. This is horribly obvious each time you see the empty
chair at the table, the unused umbrella in the hall. I remember bringing
my mother a cup of tea in bed one morning after my stepfather died and
being quite shocked at how small she looked in the big half-empty bed.
How much bigger it must have felt to her without my large, bear-like
stepfather lying there beside her.

After about a year daily life should begin to settle down and the new
routines begin to feel a bit more familiar. It is also, however, a time when
emotional support from other people will probably have stopped, and you
will have to find ways of dealing alone with resurgences of pain and grief,
which are inevitable. The period of active mourning is by no means
over – for many young people it will only just have begun.

The second year is when major changes often take place, which can
unexpectedly reawaken painful feelings you had thought were over at
last. Moving house, the remaining parent starting a new relationship,
changing jobs, all are things that may well happen in the second year of
bereavement. In the first year people usually avoid any major changes.
Instinctively you want to be still and not rock the already unsteady boat.
But after a year this may no longer be practical or necessary. Perhaps
financial pressures force a house move. Perhaps your remaining parent
finds a new partner. It is important to realize that all change involves loss
and that all change will have the power to reactivate old feelings of loss
(see Chapters 6 and 7). The best way to help yourself through these

changes is to recognize what you are losing, and to allow yourself to grieve for that loss.

Even when these changes seem positive to the outside world, the repercussions of these changes for you personally may be rather different. Allow yourself to see what you are losing and try if possible to take your feelings seriously. Pretending to yourself and other people to be coping fine now will not help you in the long run if your feelings are really much more complicated than that. It is vital not to impose a strict and arbitrary cut-off line beyond which you do not let yourself mourn. The effects of a parent's death will continue to make themselves felt for at least two years, and usually much longer. You must allow yourself this mourning time, for as long as you need it.

Anniversaries

The beginning of the second year is marked by the first anniversary of your parent's death, an occasion which many people approach with dread. Significant events in the years after a parent's death can be surprisingly hard to deal with, particularly these 'firsts'. The first Christmas, the first birthday, the first holiday: these events, and none more than the first anniversary of the death, are reminders that life is continuing for you without your parent. They are a reminder of what you have lost and of how you have changed.

Anniversaries are a particularly poignant reminder. Not only this first one, but each anniversary for many years will revive feelings and thoughts that for the rest of the year you may be able to forget. Memories of how your parent died, the place where it happened, where you were at the time, how you felt when you found out about the death, the events surrounding the death – all these are stirred up again by this annual event.

Sometimes you may feel considerable pressure from others not to mark the death of your parent, but to hurry up and forget about it. I remember one evening a few years after my father's death being invited out to dinner. I arrived early and was sitting in the kitchen chatting with my host while he finished off the cooking.

'So how are things with you?' he asked.

'Well, OK,' I replied. 'A little sad today because it's the anniversary of my father's death.'

There was a short silence, then my friend said, 'But that was ages ago. You can't keep on feeling sad about it.'

It was my turn to be surprised – and annoyed. 'I don't *want* to feel this way,' I said. 'I just *do*. I can't help it.'

However much pressure you feel to ignore the anniversary, the likelihood is that you will be aware of it anyway. This isn't so strange when you think about it: you would hardly forget your own birthday, regardless of whether other people remember it or not, and this day too is a significant one in your life. Along with your birthday, the day your parent died probably affected you more than any other day in your life so far. It is not so easy to forget a parent's death or the anniversary of it as other people sometimes suppose.

Twenty-three-year-old Michelle found herself feeling increasingly tearful in the weeks running up to the first anniversary of her father's death, and was dreading the actual day. After some thought, she decided that rather than try and just get through the day, she would take time off work and make the trip up north to where her father had lived when he was alive. Instead of trying to avoid the anniversary, Michelle decided to do the opposite: to make an event of it by going to visit her father's grave and by giving herself that day to mourn. Having made this decision, she began to feel less anxious about the day, and when it came, although the pilgrimage was not easy, she very much felt that she had done the right thing.

Fifteen-year-old Karen was not able to take charge of the anniversary of her mother's death in this way. Her family had decided that they would all go and scatter the ashes together, but could not agree where. Karen, the youngest of three children, wanted to scatter them in a park which she and her mother had often visited together, but her preference was overruled by her father and older siblings. In the end they agreed upon another park, one without personal associations, but fairly close to where they lived. They each took it in turns to throw a handful of their mother's ashes into the river that ran through the park. But when it came to Karen's turn, some people were approaching and her father hurried her. Karen was left feeling that not only had her choice of place been rejected, but that she had also been cheated of her turn to say goodbye to her mother. This was extremely painful for Karen as she already harboured a deep sense of having been allowed very little space to grieve within her family. It also heightened her identification with her mother, who, Karen believed, had killed herself because she had felt so stifled by her family. The day had gone badly wrong for Karen and her anger was intense and overwhelming. On many levels the first anniversary of her mother's death had been a profoundly negative experience for Karen. Later, however, she was able to mark the anniversary in ways that felt appropriate and meaningful to her.

Ed was 21 when his mother died. He says he is *always* aware when the anniversary is coming round. This year he and his family have decided to go back to the place in the country where his mother died, and mark the anniversary by being together that day and lighting candles in remembrance of her life. Ed says he is looking forward to it: he would rather be sharing sad and happy moments in the supportive company of friends and family, than be on his own pretending it is a day like any other.

Formal recognition of an anniversary can be very helpful, whether it is an event organized for close family, or a public memorial service. Religious communities can play an important part here too. I have already described the Jewish custom of observing the *Jahrzeit* where people light a candle at home and the name of the dead person is read out in synagogue and a special prayer said.

Sometimes, awareness of the anniversary can be deeply suppressed but nevertheless felt. At the age of 46 Hannah suddenly found herself plunged into a deep depression. Her father had committed suicide thirty years earlier when she was 19. It had never been possible to speak about his death with other members of her family and his death was never marked in any way. Hannah didn't even know when her father had died, just that it was some time in the Spring. But as a result of this sudden and profound depression, she went into counselling and began to talk about her father's death for the first time. In particular, she began to talk to other members of her family about how her father had died, and when. Through an aunt, she discovered to her astonishment that her psychological collapse coincided exactly with the date on which her father had died. Since then, she has made time to mark the anniversary of his death, to look at photos of him, and think about him, a ritual that has helped her to do the mourning and remembering she was never allowed or encouraged to do before.

Marked formally or not, anniversaries seldom go privately unmarked. I find myself very aware of the anniversary whether or not I want to be, and with time I have decided it is not worth fighting this awareness. It is far better to mark the day and use it as an occasion to remember than to try and pretend it is just a day like any other. Loss and life deserve and need to be marked. Allow yourself this day at least. Anniversaries are a valuable opportunity to remember; they can be welcomed, not denied.

Physical symptoms of grief

Grief often emerges as a physical reaction. Emotions do not exist in a vacuum, they take place in the container of the body, and very often emotional and physical reactions to a death are indistinguishable from one another. On top of the more obvious feelings you may have after a death, such as anger, guilt, sadness, irritability, fear and anxiety, you may also experience a range of physical symptoms, not just immediately after the death, for a long time after. You may well still feel and be weepy at times, easily reduced to tears or unexpectedly bursting into tears. You may be lethargic, unable to drag yourself through the day and lacking in energy. Or you may be restless, unable to concentrate, or settle to anything. A sensation of hollowness can be both a physical sensation in your stomach and an emotional emptiness. An increased risk of accidents and increased vulnerablility to illness can also still be a problem, as the Childhood Bereavement Study found.[1]

Physical symptoms are very much part of how you mourn for someone you love. It is not uncommon, for example, to imagine you have the symptoms that your dead parent had, such as tightness in the chest, or pains in the head. This may be a way to feel connected to the person who has died: physically you empathize with their situation so much that you can sometimes start to feel as you imagine they felt.

The body can also tell us things that our minds don't want to know. You may, for example, have physical symptoms that do not obviously relate to an emotion, but which nevertheless may be clues to how you are feeling. Not being able to sleep, having bad dreams and nightmares, sweating or shaky hands and nervous tics can all be physical expressions of hidden emotions. Anxiety can cause headaches, sweating, trembling or nausea. It is not uncommon to feel literally heavyhearted when you are mourning the loss of a parent, or for the area around the solar plexus to ache. To be 'sick at heart' is an old-fashioned way of saying you are deeply sad. Martin's mother died of stomach cancer when he was 19. For almost two years after her death he was gripped with a feeling of sickness in his own stomach. Martin was heart-sick and his body was telling him so. We also talk about feeling 'sick with nerves', and as Martin gradually realized with the help of a Cruse counsellor, his feeling of sickness also expressed a deep anxiety that the world was no longer a safe place for him. Twenty-year-old Tom learnt to recognize in his trembling hands his concern that he would not be able to hold things together now that his father was dead and so much responsibility for his family fell to him. Realising this consciously, made it easier for him to take practical steps to relax and share some of his worries and responsibilities.

Additional losses

Another loss or death within the first two years after a parent's death is one reason why grieving can become drawn-out and particularly difficult. Two years might have been long enough for me if my stepfather had not also died within that time.

Unfortunately, it is not uncommon for other significant losses to take place within a short space of time. In some cases this will be another death. Research has shown that widows and widowers have a higher risk of death within a year of their partner dying than unbereaved people of the same age.

Emma Judge, writing in the *Guardian*, describes how her father died of a heart attack at Easter and her mother died of cancer five months later. Her mother had already been diagnosed as terminally ill before her father's death and as Emma writes,

> Dad had been the main prop for us all while Mum was ill. He looked after her, went to all the doctors with her and comforted her. We all turned to him to know what to do. My family gathered at our house after he died; we just didn't know what to do. It was the worst day of my life.

Even if there are other relatives around to offer love and kindness and support, the death of both your parents within a short space of time is a terrible loss to bear.

Laura was an attractive, vivacious 16-year-old who'd recently started at a new school. Her mother had died when she was 7 and her father two years later. Since then she had lived with first one relation or family friend and then another. She had no emotional security or support from anyone in her life, and had had no opportunity to grieve for either of her parents or for herself. While she had clearly developed a confident and appealing external manner, her inner world was in tatters. As she relayed the tragic losses she'd suffered, she made constant jokes and wisecracks, as if seeking my approval and acceptance at any cost, even by making me laugh at her suffering. She both wanted to tell someone what had happened to her, but also was terribly afraid of the consequences of being heard. Laura had learnt from her experiences to be always on guard against further rejection. I later discovered that not one of the teachers at her new school was aware of her personal circumstances.

Maybe, however, the additional loss you have to cope with is not the death of another parent, but of a friend or relative.

Fifteen-year-old Justin had to cope with the death of his beloved grandmother and then his father within six months of each other.

Ten-year-old Katie heard that a friend of hers had been killed in a car crash and, coming soon after her father's death, this affected her very deeply even though the friend had not been an especially close one.

For twenty-year-old Nicola, it was getting pregnant and having to have an abortion that came as another intolerable loss while she was still reeling from her mother's death. In Nicola's case this second loss made it impossible for her to carry on 'coping' on her own and she sought support from a professional counsellor.

In the months following a bereavement, you will be extra-sensitive to death and to loss. It is like losing a layer of skin: you will be red-raw to anything that rubs up against you thereafter. I found I could not even stand to read reports of major disasters in the paper. Watching interviews on television with people whose relatives had been killed in the fire at the Bradford football stadium reduced me to tears. When a 19-year-old girl was murdered not far from where I live, the papers carried pictures of her family coming out of the funeral. I found their grief-worn faces unbearably moving.

Any new and direct experience of death when you are still feeling vulnerable from the first death can set you back. It reactivates the feelings of fear and vulnerability and helplessness that first engulf you when someone you love dies. You will also be sensitive to other kinds of losses, such as the loss of a job or a family home, or the loss of a parent through remarriage (see Chapters 6 and 7). All sorts of things can knock you off balance again, just as you thought you were getting yourself upright once more. In fact, loss throughout your life will tend to reactivate feelings connected with earlier losses (see Chapter 8), but it is these major losses that occur within the two-year period of mourning that can radically affect your ability to mourn and to heal. Don't underestimate the impact of these losses. They deserve to be taken seriously. And don't be too hard on yourself for being more affected than you imagine you 'should' or 'ought' to be.

Complications: when two years is not enough

William Worden's suggested two years may sound a long time, but for many people it will not be long enough. As a result of my work with young bereaved people, and from my own personal experience of being bereaved as a teenager, I know that this is nearly always the case for people who lose a parent in childhood or adolescence. At 18, I simply was not able to grieve properly. I was too young, too immature, too baffled by life and death, too insecure, too busy taking exams and leaving home. I didn't want to turn to my mother for help and it didn't occur to me to talk to friends. My father's death didn't catch up with me until I was in my mid-twenties, because it was really only then that I had the space and the emotional resources to deal with it. Not that it felt like that. It just felt as if I'd hit rock-bottom and couldn't run away from grief any longer. But now I can see that I was far more ready and able to grieve at 25 than I had been at 18.

For many people, grieving will be complicated and prolonged, but for young people in particular, the death of a parent and the two years that follow will invariably coincide with many other major changes. On top of the changes caused by death, you may be leaving home for the first time, going to college, starting a new job, taking exams, maybe even getting married or having a child. These events, however wanted and necessary, nevertheless interfere with the natural process of mourning and sometimes make it very difficult to do the necessary work of accepting a death and building a new relationship with the parent who has died. And it *is* work. Hard work, which takes time and energy and courage and honesty. It is important to recognize the additional pressures that you are having to deal with at the same time as coming to terms with death, and this coincidence of major changes may mean that for you the whole process of mourning will take much longer than two years.

Psychologists Margaret and Wolfgang Stroebe have written that 'the risk of psychiatric problems seems to be particularly high after a delay or inhibition of the initial grief response'.[2] William Worden and his colleagues at Harvard found clear evidence that young people often do not begin to experience many aspects of bereavement until two years after the death.[3] British psychotherapist, Caspar Williams, studied a group of men who'd lost parents as teenagers and found that all had gone through a period of turbulent personal crisis in their twenties or thirties, as if the full impact of their fathers' deaths could only be processed long after the event.[4] Perhaps it is time that we formulated a new framework of grieving for young people, for whom delaying grief is not just a necessary defence, but an essential strategy.

Human beings are remarkably resilient and our ability to survive and come through all sorts of appalling experiences is amazing. The majority of people, likewise, will gradually adjust and adapt to the pain of losing a parent and be able to move on with their lives. Sometimes, however, the mourning process is complicated, perhaps because of the circumstances of the death itself, or just as often by events that took place before the death of your parent, or events that took place afterwards as a direct result of their death.

Risk factors for complicated grieving

The Childhood Bereavement Study found that the number of children at risk of complicated grieving doubled in the course of the second year after a parent's death.[5] Some children may be at risk early on, but be sufficiently buffered or supported after a parent's death to adjust better as time goes on. Other children will become more at risk as time goes on, due to other factors that follow on from the death, for example family changes, family tension, and how the remaining parent is coping.

Research over the past two decades has gone a long way to identifying the risk factors in a person's life that make it much harder for them to adjust after a parent's death and which complicate the tasks of mourning.

Children at greatest risk of complicated grieving two years after a parent's death, according to William Worden, are those who:

(i) experience sudden or violent death

(ii) experience more health problems and accidents soon after death

(iii) feel increasingly sad during first year and feel closer to dead parent than living one

(iv) feel to blame for the death during second year

(v) experience high levels of concurrent stress and tension in family, including financial difficulties, frequent house moves, domestic disruption

(vi) witness passive coping style in remaining parent, or experience emotional/mental collapse of remaining parent

(vii) are in families who feel unsupported by others, including in-laws and extended family

Other risk factors include:

1. *The relationship you had with your dead person before their death*
When your relationship with the parent who dies was already difficult, this inevitably and invariably complicates the task of mourning their death. Similarly, if the relationship between your parents was chaotic, volatile and hostile, this also makes mourning a parent who has died far more difficult.

2. *Your personal history*
If you have had earlier experiences of traumatic events, or repeated loss or separation from key people in your life, this will increase the risk for complicated mourning. Exposure to domestic violence, or mental illness in one of your parents, an emotionally insecure childhood, or one in which you experienced neglectful or harsh treatment, emotionally or physically, from either of your parents before the death will predispose you to a greater likelihood of difficulty in mourning for a parent's death.

3. *Your pre-existing personality / mental health*
If you were already prone to stress, anxiety and depression, or have other pre-existing psychological difficulties, such as obsessive-compulsive disorder, bipolar disorder or borderline personality disorder, you will be additionally vulnerable emotionally and psychologically after the death of a parent.

4. *The immediate circumstances of the death*
If the body has not been recovered, or there is no definite confirmation of the death, as can be the case after a suspected murder or after a plane crash or natural disaster, the lack of closure will also greatly complicate the mourning process. Seeing a parent in great physical distress before their death is also linked to difficulties with mourning a dead parent.

5. *Domestic upheaval after the death*
Drastic changes to the routine in your household or to roles within the family after a death, prevent bereaved children getting the consistency and stability they crucially need in their daily lives after a major loss and interfere with mourning. Emotional chaos is also a risk factor. When the remaining parent becomes highly inconsistent, emotionally unavailable or is overwhelmed by depression or other psychological problems, this also deprives bereaved children and teenagers of the stability and safety they need to grieve.

6. *Poor communication after the death*
Emotional support, clear information about the bereavement and its impact on your life, and warm, consistent parenting are vital protective factors for bereaved children, as is feeling able to talk freely about your feelings and about the person who has died with friends and family. Similarly, access to information and opportunities to talk about your parent's death are also important. The absence of these puts children of all ages at greater risk of emotional and psychological problems in adjusting to the death of a parent.

It is worth asking yourself if you are, or have been, at risk from any of the above. This in turn will help you to understand the ramifications and likely repercussions of this bereavement in your life in the time ahead, and set the help you may need.

In some cases grief may feel so unbearable that the bereaved person tries to avoid grieving altogether. As Parkes and Weiss explain in *Recovery from Bereavement*, this can lead to:

1. *Unexpected-grief syndrome*
This is where the death is unexpected, sudden and untimely, and where the intense shock of the death triggers feelings of great anxiety, disbelief,

intense guilt and obligation to the person who has died. In this situation there is often a powerful desire to protect oneself from the fact of death.

2. *Ambivalent-grief syndrome*
This occurs when a person's relationship with the person who has died was characterized by ambivalence and/or conflict. There is a tendency to deny the impact of loss at first and later to feel very despairing. Initial feelings of relief and low anxiety give way to a loss of faith in relationships, guilt, self-punitive feelings and despair.

3. *Chronic-grief syndrome*
When a relationship was very over-dependent or clingy (on either side), the bereaved person may feel overcome with a sense of helplessness. Grieving can set in immediately with great intensity and continue for an unusually long time.

For people who lose a parent during their childhood or adolescence in any of the above circumstances, the risks of unexpected-grief syndrome and ambivalent-grief syndrome are increased. I first met 17-year-old Natasha ten months after her mother had died of cancer after two years of illness. Natasha had reacted to news of her mother's illness by switching off emotionally. This was the most effective way she could protect herself from the appalling shock of learning that her powerful and influential mother was going to die. She could not consciously entertain the fact of her mother's impending death, and ploughed her anxiety about her mother's illness into a programme of self-education, teaching herself everything she could about cancer. As she remarked when we met, 'I know all about how she died, but I still don't know why she died.'

Having denied that her mother was terminally ill, Natasha denied herself the chance of preparing for her death. Instead she felt angry with her mother for being weak when she was meant to be strong, deeply betrayed and abandoned. When her mother eventually died, Natasha's primary emotion was one of relief. Beyond that the feeling she was most conscious of was 'emptiness'. By the time we met she felt detached from her father and brother and was in trouble at school for disruptive behaviour. She insisted that 'nothing had changed really' since her mother's death, and was fiercely punitive of any lapse from her self-imposed stance of emotional imperviousness. She explained that she didn't want to think about her mother's death because there were more productive ways of spending her time. Yet not far beneath this tough exterior, there were clear signs of a terrified and vulnerable child, whose mother's death had torn the core out of her life.

Sometimes you may experience physical symptoms and emotions that are not easy to understand. When the cause is particularly complicated or deeply suppressed, for whatever reasons, you may find that you are projecting your feelings out into the world, rather than experiencing them directly. It is as if you have turned the world, or sometimes just one aspect of it, into a great white screen, on to which you then throw the image of your most hidden feelings and fears.

David was 21 when his father died. They had had a close but complicated relationship. Even while his father was alive, David often felt that his father was overambitious for him, unduly critical and impossible to please. After his father's death, he became obsessed with cleanliness, washing his hands over and over again in the course of the day. He also became obsessed with the hidden danger of asbestos, convinced that the rooms he was in were full of poisonous asbestos fumes which were seeping into him. On one occasion he became so panic-stricken about this invisible threat that he rang his sister and pleaded with her to come to his flat to check it over for asbestos. A professional company was called in. Needless to say, there was no asbestos in his flat.

What David was projecting on to the world was his own secret fear that something in him was bad and destructive. Secretly he feared that this hidden 'poison', which he sensed all around him, was already inside him. The more he unconsciously worried that he was in fact the source of this poison, the more frantically he tried to find it in some source outside himself. The 'poison' he so feared was several things: unexpressed anger that he had often felt towards his father for being so critical of him; the irrational fantasy that this anger had somehow killed his father; and the profound fear that his father had been right to be so critical and that he, David, was a bad person, not deserving of approval or praise; capable, in fact, of terrible destruction.

Fiona had a milder form of the same type of deeply hidden feelings and fears. After her mother's death she became very sensitive to 'bad' smells, imagining she could detect excrement or sewage everywhere she went. After a few months the acute awareness of unpleasant smells faded back to normal, but Fiona began to realize that her obsession with bad smells recurred whenever she was feeling anxious, worried or under pressure. With the help of a therapist, whom she was seeing to help with her feelings after her mother's death, Fiona eventually remembered that as a child she had suffered from the same preoccupation with smells around the time when her parents had divorced and her father left home. For Fiona, imagining that she could smell something rotten and bad was a way of expressing her own buried childhood fear that she herself was the bad, rotten presence which first her father and later her mother had not wanted to be near. It was her own fear that she was not good, not nice to be near, that she could smell, a classic example of the kind of 'magical thinking' that young children are vulnerable to after traumatic losses, as I described earlier.

For both David and Fiona these complicated reactions were triggered, though not directly caused by grief, and took a long time to untangle. Though not always in such extreme forms, most of us will have childhood fears of some kind which in adulthood may require sorting out, looking at and dealing with. Often this process involves learning to see your parents and yourself more objectively, more kindly, in order to understand why they behaved as they did and why you reacted as you did. The trouble for those who are still young when parents die is that it makes this process much more difficult. Young children are especially at risk from these kind of 'crossed wires'. Seven-year-old Anna, whose mother had died suddenly in a sailing accident, began refusing to bath in the evening and at the same time started wetting the bed at night. Her father was soon exasperated and exhausted by this extra work of changing and washing sheets, and Anna was in turn frightened by her father's annoyance, fearing he too might leave her for being 'naughty'. The whole business was causing them both great distress. Eventually Anna was referred to a therapist who, through gentle play therapy and talk, uncovered what Anna was expressing through bed-wetting. Her fear of bath time related to her anxiety that she too might drown and die, while her bed-wetting revealed a deeply repressed longing to be under water and reunited with her mother.

One of the problems about losing a parent in childhood or adolescence is that it's easy to get stuck emotionally and psychologically at the point at which they died. Even though your parent is no longer alive to help, you still need to find ways of continuing to develop the *adult* relationship that you and your parent would have had had they lived. Not only do you have fewer inner resources to deal with what's happened and make sense of it when you are young, you are not yet ready to be independent at a psychological and emotional level. Research in the field of psychology and neuroscience has shown how from the earliest months of life, our identity is formed in relation to those closest to us. In *Why Love Matters*, psychotherapist Sue Gerhardt draws on findings from both these fields to show how in the first few months of life our brains continue to develop in response to the care we receive from the adults in our lives. If we receive very inadequate care at this stage, for example, we can become over- or under-sensitive to stress, and more prone to anxiety and depression throughout our lives as a result. During childhood and adolescence, our identity continues to be shaped negatively and positively by those around us, and most of all by our parents or other key carers. As we move through childhood, parents provide us with a vital and fundamental mirror. We see ourselves reflected in them, we mimic and learn from what we see them doing, how we see them behaving and responding, and as we get older, we begin to make decisions about whether we accept or reject what we see in that mirror. The teenage years are a critical time for this kind of testing, rejecting and adapting of ourselves in relation to the parental figures in our lives. The death of a parent, however, means that this normal process is halted in its tracks.[6] The mirror is suddenly gone. The impact of this can range from distressing to disastrous, depending on other factors in our lives, but many people bereaved as children or teenagers often say later that they feel as if something in them stopped growing or developing at that point. They feel they got stuck at the age when the mirror vanished. Outwardly, physically, we continue to grow and mature, but inside, time may have stopped, because the much-needed and entirely taken-for-granted reflection that our parents provide has stopped.

There are several ways to reduce and cope with this problem. The first and perhaps most important is to recognize that other people now have to be that mirror for you. Sometimes your remaining parent will be able to help you with that, not only by providing their continuing love and support, but just as importantly by sharing memories of your dead parent, and giving you space to talk about them and learn about them, as parents and as people. Our feelings about and relationship with a living parent continue to change throughout our lives and it's the same with a parent who has died. You need to be able to update your sense of who they were and how they influenced you, for good and bad, as you move through your life. When a close friend of mine discovered she had terminal cancer at the age of 38, she asked what she could do to help her four children, then aged 7, 10, 12 and 14. We decided to record her life story, so that after she died, her children could still listen to her voice, and find answers to questions about her that they might need as they grew up. We talked about her childhood, her relationships with her parents and siblings, her experiences at school and university, how she met their father, how she felt about getting married and becoming a parent, how she felt about dying and having to leave them. These were not things her children wanted to know about when she died, but as they grew up, these were likely to be exactly the kind of things they would want to have asked her. It took considerable courage and foresight for my friend to record her memories and experiences in this way, but her eldest child, now in her twenties, has already begun to listen to the recording and finds it very helpful.

If you can't get answers as directly as this, you can still ask other adults in your life who knew your parent. Sometimes, that won't be possible, in which case it is a conversation you need to have with yourself, or perhaps with the help of a counsellor or therapist. Finding ways to continue to have a connection with your parent is not just ok, it's a really important part of continuing to grow and develop yourself, not only as a child, but as a person.

Getting support

You may well find yourself needing more support than you are getting from friends and family, especially if you are still struggling with depression or anxiety in the second year after a parent's death or beyond. As the sociologist Geoffrey Gorer wrote after carrying out his classic research into bereavement and mourning in Britain in the 1960s: 'Human beings mourn in response to grief, and if mourning is denied outlet, the result will be suffering, either psychological or physical or both.' Given how little recognition there is of the needs of people whose parents have died, it is not improbable that your grief will be denied outlet, at some stage and to some degree, and this may cause you problems somewhere along the line.

When a child needs professional help

Sometimes professional help is necessary and invaluable. In his book *Children and Grief*, William Worden has identified ten key indicators that a bereaved child is in need of professional help:

1. If child has persistent difficulty talking about dead parent, e.g. can't bear to talk about dead parent or be in same room as people who are doing so
2. If aggressive behaviour persists or takes increasingly destructive forms into and beyond the second year after death
3. If anxiety persists beyond first year after death, and/or gets worse, leading to clinging, phobic behaviour around separations, nightmares and other anxiety related behaviour
4. If somatic symptoms persist beyond first year, or if symptoms develop some time after the death, or if pre-existing symptoms worsen markedly after the death
5. If sleep disturbances continue beyond the first few months after death
6. If there are marked or persistent changes in eating patterns
7. If there is marked social withdrawal beyond first few months after death

8. If there are school difficulties or serious academic reversal during second year or after
9. If there is persistent and pervasive self-blame or guilt, which are symptoms of clinical depression
10. If there is self-destructive behaviour, or suicidal thoughts

These kinds of behaviours and thoughts are what Worden calls 'red flags'. They are ways for the child to express needs that are not being met, and are therefore indicators that the child is struggling and in need of attention and support in particular areas. Understanding what these behaviours are expressing is therefore extremely important, whether you are the child in question, or whether you are an adult trying to support a grieving young person. These 'red flags' include:

Expressing insecurity – signal that child needs greater sense of safety/reassurance

Expressing feelings of abandonment – leads to self-fulfilling prophecy of being unloved – signal that child's needs for safety/security need prioritizing

Provoking punishment – this can be a way to feel secure / noticed / contained – signal that child needs to feel more secure / needs more consistent parenting / boundary setting

Subtly alienating others – this can be an attempt to prevent future losses – signal that fear for safety of self/others is acute, and indicates need for reassurance that relationships are safe

Rejecting others – this can be a way to avoid the pain of future losses – signal that trauma of loss has led to fear of forming new attachments and indicates need for reassurance and help with trust and positive thinking to believe it is safe to make attachments to others

Hyperactivity – this can be a way to counter personal death anxieties – signal that anxiety has become destructive and indicates need for help with managing/reducing stress

Externalizing internal feelings of grief – signal that child needs help managing internal feelings to avoid acting out in destructive ways.

Awareness of the needs of bereaved young people in particular has greatly increased in recent years. You may be lucky enough to have adults around you who *do* understand what you are going through. But if not, a number of organizations now exist that provide support specifically for bereaved children and teenagers. Older teenagers and young adults are more likely to find themselves in the position of having to go out and find support for themselves. After a parent's death this may feel like the last thing you want or are able to do. The idea of making yourself more vulnerable than you already are by going and talking to someone can be really frightening. You may feel you will be stirring up painful feelings that are best left alone. It is essential that you are straight with yourself. Are you really OK? Are you really managing without anyone to talk to or share your feelings with? After my father and step-father died, I became very aware of how little support was actually available for young people like me, who were trying to establish their own lives at the same time as coming to terms with the death of a parent. My tutors were sympathetic, but left it to me to go to them – something I did not feel able to do. Nor did I want to talk to the university helpline, largely because it was run by students and I didn't think they would understand what I was going through. The university did have a counselling service, but again, the onus was on me to make an appointment and get myself there. I would think about it when I was feeling really low, but then I'd think: 'Well, leave it a day and I might feel a bit better in the morning.' By the next morning I wouldn't feel much better, but I would have persuaded myself I was making a fuss about nothing, that there was nothing anyone could say or do to help anyway. Looking back, I think I was actually terrified of talking to anyone in case it made me feel even worse than I already did. Avoiding getting support was a way of avoiding facing the pain of loss, avoiding feeling any more vulnerable.

However frightening the idea of talking about your grief and sorrow and loss may seem, is it really worse than carrying it around in the back of your mind like a great dark shadow the whole time, hoping it will have gone the next time you look, but never quite daring to look in case it hasn't?

The idea of talking to a stranger may seem daunting, but it can be an immense relief to share what you are going through with someone qualified to help, and experienced in the painful, lonely ways of bereavement. There is nothing to be gained from loneliness. Finding an understanding person to talk to will make you feel far less isolated, far less different than you may imagine you are. A school or college counsellor, or a specially trained bereavement counsellor or therapist, will certainly appreciate and be knowledgeable about the effect of a major bereavement on your life, and the simple act of talking to other people really can help. While you have not been through this experience before, other people have, and they will understand that talking helps. They will not consider it a sign of weakness, as you may fear it is.

Don't be put off seeing a professional by worries about what other people may say or think. It's you that counts. Don't be afraid to seek out understanding support whenever you need it – once a month, once a week, once a day. It doesn't matter. It is not shameful to need support. If you want support but don't want to talk to someone face-to-face, there are also a number of phone helplines you can call, as well as online support (see p. 210–21).

There are other ways, apart from talking, to relieve the burden of troubling thoughts and feelings. After her mother's death, the main source of comfort for Ruth was her painting. She found she could channel much of her bewilderment and sorrow into art. 'I didn't have anyone to talk to about how I was feeling,' she recalls, 'so it just all came out in my painting. The things appearing on the canvasses were pretty strange, but it was a really important outlet.' Producing something creative out of such a deadening negative experience helped give Ruth a sense of her own life continuing, of the reality of her existence when everything seemed so unreal.

Other people have found comfort in playing the piano, writing short stories or a journal, doing pottery or sewing. At Winston's Wish in Gloucestershire, an organization that works with bereaved families, children are encouraged to make Film Script stories about how their parents died to help them express and make sense of what has happened.[7] Film Script stories are a series of pictures that tell a story, a bit like a comic strip. This is a good way to order events in your own mind, and is particularly helpful if you are experiencing repeated unwanted thoughts about a parent's death. Once the child has drawn their Film Script, telling the story of what life was like before their parent died, what happened when they died, and how life has changed since, they roll up the script and put it away. The act of doing this physically makes it easier for children then to say 'stop' to the unwanted pictures playing in their heads. It helps put the child in charge of his or her thoughts. Ten-year-old John and his father were out cycling when his father was knocked over and killed. In the weeks after his father's death, John suffered from recurrent flashbacks to his death. By making a Film Script story about how his father had died, John was able to take some control over these thoughts, which came as an immense relief.

Doing something, *making* something out of the dreadful nothingness of a loved parent's absence is a way of filling the physical, emotional and psychological void left by their death.

Some form of expressive activity in this bewildering time can help to ease the gaping emptiness that you may feel. When it is connected with your emotions at a deep level – as painting or writing or music are – such activities can also help to maintain the links with your parent's influence and presence, and their importance to you. To have this, when you may feel that you are under pressure to erase your parent from your life, or when you feel troubled by painful thoughts and feelings about their death, can be extremely helpful.

Key needs of parentally bereaved children

Struggling with loss is normal whatever your age. But children and young people especially need the help and support of adults around them as they adjust. From the time of the death and for *at least* the first two years after, bereaved children and teenagers need the following:

1. Information: children need to be given clear and comprehensible information at time of death and after to minimize risk of feeling anxious and unsafe.
2. Involvement in mourning rituals: children need to be involved and included in preparations for the death and for the funeral, and to have their views and needs about the funeral taken into account, heard and respected. Similarly, they need to be included in rituals around anniversaries of parent's death, birthdays, and other significant days.
3. Freedom from blame: children need to know they are not to blame. This is especially important for 4–5-year-olds, who are most at risk of 'magical thinking', believing they are culpable for the death.
4. Security: children need consistency, stability and physical and emotional affection in order to help them recover their sense of internal and external safety. Disruptions and major changes need to be kept to a minimum.
5. Validation: children need to have their fears, fantasies and questions heard and respected, not dismissed or minimized. Listeners do not need to be parents, can be friends, teachers, counsellors or other relatives.
6. Permission to grieve: children need to know that strong emotions are a normal part of mourning; in particular, sadness, anxiety, fear, guilt and anger. They need to have their own feelings of grief acknowledged and respected, and to be given space and permission to grieve in the way they want for as long as they need.
7. Normality: children need to continue with activities appropriate to their age – to play, to go out with friends, to be lazy, to be selfish.

Bereaved children don't need to lose their childhood in addition to their parent.

8. Positive role models: children need people around them to model effective and active grieving, i.e. who can feel and tolerate strong feelings of sadness, anger, missing, but not be overwhelmed by them.

9. Opportunities to remember: children need opportunities to remember their dead parent not just after death, but continuously throughout life, through memories, shared reflections and conversations about dead person.

10. Permission to continue the bond: children need permission and regular opportunities to reappraise their dead parent and update their knowledge and relationship with them for as long as they need.

As far as possible try to be patient and honest with yourself about what you are feeling and thinking, and do try to have faith in the fact that you *will* find a meaning for this tragic event, that you *will* be able to make a place in your life both for your dead parent and for the fact of his or her death. Try to remember that it does take time and that the best person to give you permission to take that time is you.

In the first two years there will be moments when it may seem extraordinarily hard to believe that you are getting used to the death of your parent, that depression and feelings of hopelessness may actually be signs that you are fairly far down the road to recovery (whatever 'recovery' means to you). Try and *trust* that this is so, however unlikely it may seem.

These weeks, months and years without the parent you love and need can seem unbearable, but usually with time you find that somehow you have borne them. Be kind and gentle with yourself in the meantime and try not to look too far ahead; just take one step at a time. The night is always darkest, it is said, in the hour before the dawn.

6

CHANGES AND LOSSES

The private kind

Every entrance is also an exit. Every gain is also a loss.
Audrey T. McCollum

A parent's death will nearly always be the catalyst for a whole series of changes in your life, internally and externally. It can often seem as if nothing is left untouched by death. And on top of the vast change caused by your parent's death alone, all these extra changes can sometimes feel unbearable. The gaps left in your daily life after a parent's death are hard to tolerate at first. You miss the voice in the hall, the face at the door, the Sunday morning phone call, the kiss at bedtime. And then gradually you and your family begin to shift and rearrange yourselves to fill those gaps. Somebody else makes supper or washes it up; somebody else takes charge of emptying the bins or putting out the milk bottles. Somebody else now takes the car to be serviced or weeds the garden. Somebody else buys the newspaper on Sunday mornings.

Sometimes these changes make life easier: it can be reassuring for life to start functioning again, for the chaos after a death to be coming to an end. These daily routines and rituals can keep you going, renew your confidence in the world and in life, distract you from the sadness you are feeling. But sometimes these changes can be distressing, making you feel that the person you love has been easily dismissed, replaced, their death forgotten. Sometimes the changes do not make things 'as before', but instead underline how very different life is now.

In our house daily life hardly changed at all after my father's death because I didn't live with him, but after my stepfather's death things at home changed dramatically. My mother now had a full-time job, and much of the household work, previously done by my stepfather, was simply left undone. Mealtimes were no longer friendly, civilized events, but rushed and haphazard affairs, everyone eating in silence and hurrying back to whatever they'd been doing before. No one seemed to be communicating. We all just lived in our own little bubbles alongside one another. It was hard for my mother to maintain much discipline or routine without her husband to help; regular bedtimes went out of the window along with any kind of rules about friends coming round. Far from feeling sympathy for my mother for having so much to worry about, I felt angry with her for not protecting us from so much unwanted change. I wanted things as they had been. As a parent myself, I have more understanding and sympathy now for what she must have been going through. At the time, I just felt angry and critical of her.

It is *essential* to make changes in your life, to take risks, to try new things, but it is equally important – and I talk as the fool who invariably rushed in – to look at the *loss* involved in change, as well as the gain. It is important to expect and allow time to mourn what is being lost as a result of these changes, and expect and allow past feelings of loss to re-emerge. To lose things that matter to you is to lose a little part of yourself; when you have already lost a large part of yourself through your parent's death, even quite small later losses can reopen the old wounds. On top of the pain of the new loss you feel all over again the pain of the old one. You need to work out what it is you are losing and mourn for it.

A double bereavement

For people in their teens and twenties, coping with the loss and change that comes with a bereavement is particularly challenging as it comes on top of the many losses and changes that already mark the passage from childhood to adulthood. Getting used to a parent's death involves changes and loss in the way we view ourselves and the world; so does making the transition from childhood to adulthood.

In her book, *Counselling Young People*, E. Doolan describes adolescence as a period of transition similar in many respects to bereavement; one which involves losing aspects of yourself and mourning for that loss. Mood swings, anger, guilt, depression, impatience and impetuousness are all emotional states common to the bereaved and to the adolescent. Her analogy highlights one of the major difficulties for people whose parents die when they are still young: you are *already* going through a kind of bereavement, losing parts of yourself and the people around you. A parent's death at the same time is a double blow, an additional loss and shock in a time of already considerable shock and loss.

You may *want* to leave home, you may *want* to go to college, you may *want* to get married, you may *want* to move into your own flat. All these things you may genuinely want and need to do, but they will involve loss as well as gain. If you can spare enough time to anticipate what you will be losing, it will come as less of a shock, and be easier to deal with.

Modern society allows ever less time for things: trains and cars are getting faster; book jackets must grab our attention in a matter of seconds; emails and mobile phones mean we are expected to respond instantly to other people; we spend increasingly less time cooking and cleaning because gadgets and inventions do these things for us. As a result of all this timesaving and speeding-up, we are free to get on with doing more things more quickly with the rest of our time! But adjusting to major change won't be hurried along by modern technology: it takes as much time as it needs. After a bereavement, a significant event in your life, like moving house, leaving your family, or starting your first job, the period of adjustment will be correspondingly more complicated, lengthy and subtle.

Private change and public change

There are basically two kinds of change and it can be helpful to separate the two. The first are the changes that come as a direct result of your parent's death, and in its immediate wake. These changes involve losses which may be vividly evident to you, but may not be so obvious to anyone else, such as a loss of routine, a loss of confidence, a sense of having lost your youth, and, perhaps most painful of all, the feeling that you have lost your living parent too.

The second kind of changes are those that come as a matter of course, but which are particularly hard for you to handle because of your parent's death, such as moving house, changing job, or ending a relationship. These changes are clearly visible to everyone, but what is not always evident to other people is that you may experience these changes not as positive or neutral changes in your life, but as painful losses.

This chapter and the next look at both of these kinds of change in turn, and at the losses they may involve.

Changing roles

One of the most difficult changes that takes place after a parent dies is the change in roles within the family. Such change is often extremely uncomfortable. You may find yourself mothering your mother or being the 'wife' to your father, or parenting younger siblings. Being the brave one, or the weak one, or the one who 'is coping marvellously' – any one of these roles can be a straitjacket at a time when you need space not restrictions. It is not very helpful to be cast in these roles and often they can make it impossible for you to know or act on what you really think and feel.

Role changes of this kind are always difficult to cope with, and if your parent dies when you are still a child or a teenager, they can be particularly problematic. Teenagers, for instance, are already trying to negotiate changes from one role to another whether a parent dies or not, and it is a slow, complicated process. It takes time to find ways to be the grown-up son who can take care of himself, not the little boy whose shoelaces were always undone. It takes time to discover how to be the grown-up daughter who knows perfectly well not to take lifts from strangers. It takes time to learn how to be an adult 'child' in relation to your parents, to see them as people not just parents. This same process is happening with siblings: trying to end fifteen years of unbroken warfare with brothers and sisters is not easy, neither is making the change from bossy older sibling to friend. Outside your family you are also taking on new roles; no longer just a child, you may now also be a wage-earner, homeowner, car-driver, credit card-holder, lover, maybe even a parent yourself.

It can take years and years to negotiate these changes in the way you see yourself and the way you are seen by family and friends. But when a parent dies, there is no time any more. Suddenly you must be able to act as an adult. There is no room anymore for the part of you that still wants to be 15 or 8 or 4. You lose a part of yourself and you lose it suddenly.

Often you will not only find you have to take responsibility for yourself as never before, but you may well be taking responsibility for other people too, such as brothers, sisters, the remaining parent, or even friends. Their needs will not always tally with yours. One year after the death of a parent, teenage girls frequently report less free time and time with friends because of additional household responsibilities, which is often a source of some resentment.[1]

When her mother died, Paula became a kind of parent to her younger siblings. She had to take them to school, make their tea, talk to them about problems with their teachers, help them with their homework. And she disliked this role intensely. 'I was their sister, I didn't *want* to be a parent to them,' she recalls. In the long term it proved impossible to be a sister and a parent-figure: 'Years of quizzing them, in my capacity of pseudo-parent, about schoolwork, life-plans, smoking and drinking, sex and contraception, made a gulf between us. In some ways I lost them as siblings when our mum died.'

One of the most moving letters I have received from a reader came from a 17-year-old girl who told me how she had become a kind of surrogate partner to her mother after her father's death, and how that had affected her in the long run.

> At the beginning of my final year at school, my father committed suicide whilst my mother and I were out for two hours at an audition for a musical. At the age of sixteen I was left devastated. The person who was so responsible and loving, and a vital part of my life left a wife and daughter totally stunned, shocked, distraught … I can't find the words to explain the feelings. I completed my year at school, meanwhile helping Mum re-establish her business. She had no one else to talk to and so I became her sounding board. Throughout the following months I blocked out all my own emotions. I couldn't have coped otherwise. I was exhausted physically and emotionally but I wouldn't allow myself to cry and grieve.

Suppressing her own emotions in this way enabled Chloe to support her mother and to live up to her own image of herself as a 'good daughter', but beneath the surface her feelings of anger and betrayal, as well as despair and loneliness, were building up. Eventually she recognized that instead of simply coping with her father's death, she needed, as she put it, to 'face and assess his death; to accept that I have lost something enormous in my life, that I am allowed to hurt, and to gradually try to heal myself.'

The oldest child in a family is usually the most at risk of finding him or herself with a new and often burdensome role after a parent dies. But sometimes this role falls to a younger sibling if, for example, she is the only girl in the family and the mother has died, or the only boy after the father has died. Whatever your rank in the family this 'shoe-filling' can create real difficulties: it is deeply confusing to have to 'become' your mother or father at exactly the time when you are trying to work out who you are in your own right.

Saul was only 10 when his father died, but the effects of the role he had to play after his father's death lasted throughout his teens and twenties. The youngest of six children and the only son in an Orthodox Jewish family, Saul found himself, at the age of 10, both the man of the household and the baby. His mother's expectations of him were high. He had to be not only her little boy, but husband to her, and father to his older sisters. Furthermore the family's income was dramatically reduced after his father's death and they were forced to move to a much smaller house. As the youngest child and only boy, Saul had to sleep in the living room until he was 13. His father's death had at one stroke deprived him of childhood, stability and privacy. From then on Saul was literally and symbolically in the public eye, the focus of everyone's attention. At 15 he left home. At 19 he left the country. These dramatic breaks were the only way he felt able to escape the pressure of the roles his father's death had left him to fill. He had to cut himself off from his home and country altogether, reject them and make it impossible for his family to reach him, in order to find the space to live his own life. He had to have an ocean and a continent between him and his closest relations before he felt far enough away to live his life for himself, able to be who he wanted to be, not act out a series of roles.

Penny's mother died when she was 15; she had two younger brothers and very much took over running the household. Despite the fact that she was still very young herself, Penny became mother and wife to her brothers and father. At 17 she abandoned her A levels and at 18 she got married. Within three years she had two children of her own. Ten years later she 'flipped', as she puts it. She left her husband, went to live abroad, and for a while became seriously anorexic: she simply rejected wholesale the responsible adult role she had been forced into so early. Being a mother was something she had done without thinking, but as her own children got older and less dependent on her, she began to see how little mothering she had had herself, how she wanted and needed to be young and free. She had to break out of her own marriage and family in order to begin to put together an adult life at her own pace.

Sarah, on the other hand, took on her father's role of being the responsible one in the family. After his death, she put on a lot of weight, became very serious and anxious, and unconsciously even began to adopt her dead father's posture and walk. At 17 she looked bowed down with the weight on her shoulders. Her family didn't object: it was nice for them to feel there was still somebody around with their best interests at heart; it made them feel somehow that their father/husband was still around. 'She's so like her father,' everyone said, as if this were a natural and good way to be. It wasn't until Sarah left home that she realized what had happened and that it was *not* her responsibility to look after the entire family. She realized that her relationship with her father had centred on his care for her, and that was what she missed. *Being* him didn't help her to come to terms with *missing* him, nor did it help her to incorporate his importance to her into her own life in a way that did not actually prevent her living it.

In some cases, a parent's death can leave you *without* a role. Michael was 14 when his father killed himself by taking an insulin overdose. There had been a lot of conflict within the family and his father had suffered from depression in the past. Michael had been his father's confidante, the one his father talked to about what he was feeling and thinking. This gave Michael an important role in a turbulent household. He was the go-between, the peacemaker. After his father died, he was left struggling with a profound sense of failure, but also without a clear place in the family. He became very depressed himself, and began to experience the same troubling thoughts and feelings his father had once described to him. With the help of a bereavement counsellor, he slowly began to understand the reasons why this was happening to him. He began to understand that by feeling similar emotions to those his father had experienced he could continue to feel close to his father. Michael also began to see how merging their identities was a way of trying to protect himself from his own grief and the sense of having failed to prevent his father's death. Within the family as a whole, there was a further incentive for Michael to 'become' his father: the causes of the conflict between his parents had not been resolved at the time of his father's death and, by representing his father's position, Michael was both holding out the possibility of resolution and also protecting his mother from confronting the fact that, now her husband was dead, resolution was impossible.

Stepping into your dead parent's shoes is often an unconscious action, and you realize only much later what has happened. For a while it can seem to lessen the pain of your loss by minimizing the impact of your parent's absence. Ultimately, however, it cannot protect you from the impact of the death. The gap left in your life has to be faced at some point and 'being' your parent cannot indefinitely prevent the pain of having lost them.

The importance of gender

It is these shifts in roles within the family that probably begin to make you aware of what specifically has been lost since your mother or father died. Much recent research shows that the death of a mother affects a family differently from the death of a father, and also that the ways in which sons and daughters react to and cope with a parent's death differ. The experiences of a daughter losing a mother are not exactly the same as a son losing a mother, any more than a daughter's reaction to a father's death is the same as a son's. The British bereavement support organization Cruse publishes two leaflets entitled *My Mother Died* and *My Father Died* in recognition of the different roles a parent plays and the different impact of their death. Although gender stereotypes are slowly changing within families, mothers and fathers still tend to take on different roles within the home, which means that when one of them dies, his or her role will be very obviously vacant – and not necessarily easy for the remaining parent to fill.

When a mother dies

Mothers in most families still tend to be the parent who provides children with most day-to-day emotional and practical support. Losing a mother can therefore leave many children with a chronic lack of emotional intimacy and emotional care at exactly the time that their need for it is particularly acute. A mother's death in this way can make a bad situation a great deal worse. A mother's death is more likely to lead to dramatic practical changes in how the household runs on a daily basis, and on who does what within the family. Children whose mothers die report most difficulty in talking about their dead parent and expressing their feelings in general.[2]

Part of the problem is that many fathers cope with their grief in ways that are not always helpful to their children. Men are less inclined to show their feelings, and less likely to encourage their children to share and express theirs. Fathers also have a harder time adjusting to life as a single parent and managing sole responsibility for day-to-day household tasks and routines. The Childhood Bereavement Study found that very few fathers reduced their work hours after their wives died, which meant they were not physically around for their children. For fathers, this return to their normal work routine was an important coping strategy. Work was a place for them to escape and forget. As one father was honest enough to admit: 'I increased my hours to keep busy and to make up for the lost hours during the last weeks of [my wife's] life. I didn't even think of the kids. It took me 6 months before I was aware that they had needs too.'[3]

Fathers are more likely to adopt a 'business as usual' approach to life after a mother's death, not only for themselves but also for their children, and they are often less sensitive to their children's need to adjust gradually. Another father in the Childhood Bereavement Study said with regret: 'It took me almost a year before I realized that they lost their mother. It wasn't only that I lost my wife.'[4]

With less experience of managing the emotional side of family life before the death, fathers often take longer to adjust to this new role afterwards, which increases their children's sense of isolation and lack of emotional support. Studies have shown that bereaved children of all ages very much benefit from stable routines, consistent discipline and boundary-setting, and good communication – all things that many bereaved fathers struggle with in the period after a mother's death.[5] It's not that fathers don't worry about the impact of the death on their children; they do, but they are much less likely than mothers to discuss their feelings with their children, or to help and encourage their children to talk about their own feelings and thoughts.

Conflict within the family after a mother's death is also more likely to be a problem, particularly between teenage girls and their fathers.[6] After her mother's death, 16-year-old Janie found herself constantly fighting with her father, in part because of what she saw as 'the countless stupid rules' he set about what time she had to be in and how often she was allowed out. 'He expected me to help around the house the whole time as if I was now the mother, but at the same time he treated me like a complete kid.' With the benefit of hindsight, Janie can see that her father was as out of his depth as she was. She can also see that she was in some ways testing her father by fighting with him. 'I think I was really scared that he was going to die too and I was trying to find out if he was there for me, if I could trust him to be there, not abandon me.'

Over time, most fathers do become more sensitive to their children's needs, more aware that they need to be available and supportive to their children. In the Childhood Bereavement Study one father, who had buried himself in work at first, gradually realized that he needed to be home for supper, and needed to relieve his eldest son of the burden of being a parent to the younger ones: 'I told my oldest boy he was not his kid brother's father, that was my job and I was here to do it.'[7]

When a mother dies, what goes with her very often is the secure organized base of your world, emotionally and physically: there is no one now to ensure the sheets are washed, the cupboards stocked, the bread fresh, your games-kit ready, your school shirts ironed. There is no one who knows the minute details of your life, the names of your friends, the size of your shoes, the last time you had a dental check-up. These are all roles that mothers still perform far more often than fathers, intimately involved as they are with the day-to-day running of your life. You may not even have been fully aware of your mother doing and knowing these things, until she is no longer there.

But it's not only practical care that can vanish when a mother dies. Women are, in general, much better at reading their children's moods than fathers. They are more sensitive to cues that their children are upset, worried, cross, down-in-the-dumps, and often more skilled in negotiating domestic conflict. Research on brain differences between men and women has found that women are hard-wired for this kind of emotional responsiveness, having far more receptors for decoding facial expressions than men.[8] If you are a boy whose mother has died, then you may well feel that the caring, warm, supportive, nurturing, accepting element of your life has gone. For a girl, a mother's death may mean not only those things have gone, but also an ally, a companion, a friend and adviser as she navigates the path through sexual maturation into adulthood. The impact of a mother's death is also affected by your age, which is why children within the same family can react and adjust differently. In this respect, older children seem to have particular difficulties after the death of a mother, especially in their relationship with their remaining parent.[9]

For very young children, the need for the kind of consistent responsive care that is still normally provided by a mother is all-important and can be very hard for fathers to provide, particularly if they are having to earn the family income as before. Mothering still tends to mean something different from fathering and, the younger the child, the truer that is. Faced with the total disappearance of their mother, babies and toddlers will be anxious at first and, if not responded to with a great deal of love and sensitivity, they can eventually become despairing and then emotionally shut down. This may be why younger children seem to cope better with the death of a father, than the death of a mother.

When a father dies

When a father dies, mothers may in general be better at helping their children process the emotional loss by providing opportunities to talk and share feelings, but of course that will very much depend on the mother. One study of British teenage boys who'd lost fathers found that for these boys none of the mothers had encouraged expression of feeling. 'The pervasion of the British stiff upper lip mentality with regards to expression of grief [meant that none of these boys had] a real opportunity to emote or process their grief within the family.'[10] As one of the interviewees in this study put it: 'I remember being very tearful [at the funeral] but feeling the need not to show it! I wasn't going to break down in tears ... it was a struggle but that was the example set by mother.'[11]

Depression is common in both mothers and fathers after the death of their spouse. One study found that 56 per cent of parents were assessed as depressed four months after the death, and 40 per cent were still depressed at the end of the first year. Women were more likely to remain depressed than men, and poorer households had higher risk of depressed mothers.[12] Bereaved mothers can be more obviously felled by their own feelings of loss, and are more vulnerable to mental health difficulties than bereaved fathers.[13] This in turn can be the cause of considerable additional anxiety in their children. The remaining parent's mental and emotional resilience has been shown to be closely linked to how you yourself will cope and adjust, and seeing your mother overwhelmed by grief is inevitably distressing and stressful. The Child Bereavement Study found, however, that even depressed mothers were more sensitive to their children's needs than the fathers. Many of the mothers were also able to make significant changes to their working lives, either leaving work altogether or reducing their hours to work part time, in order to be more available to their children. Partly this reflected the fact that men were more likely to have been insured for illness and death, giving the woman more financial flexibility after a death.[14]

Children of all ages are very sensitive to how their remaining parent is feeling and coping, and are distressed by irritability, distractedness, unhappiness, and impatience in their living parent. Where there is a lot of conflict with the remaining parent, children are more likely to become withdrawn, and show higher levels of anxiety and depression, as well as aggression, acting out, and higher rate of accidents.

Your relationship with your father before his death plays an important part in how you adjust afterwards. A study at Kansas State University in America of twenty female students whose fathers had died found that 70 per cent described their father as someone they had felt very close to before their death. The students who seemed to be coping best with their bereavements were the ones who had found a positive way of continuing their relationship with their father as a welcome, helpful presence in their lives. Those women who had tried to cut off from their fathers, or who felt troubled by memories of them, were also more bothered by what their father's death meant and its significance in their lives.[15]

The death of a father can leave both boys and girls without an important guide, protector, friend, comforter and role model. Your father was maybe the person you played sport with, or the person who helped you with your homework. You and he may have shared a hobby you loved, or maybe what you miss is something as simple as skimming stones together. Psychotherapist Caspar Williams gives this very moving account of losing his father when he was a teenager:

> When I was fifteen, my father died. It was May 1981 and I had just returned to boarding school for the start of the summer term. I had known that my father was going into hospital for extensive surgery to remove a duodenal ulcer. My parents played down the seriousness of this and I was assured he was making a good recovery following his five hour operation. It came as a complete shock when my father died a week later from a blood clot induced heart attack. At the time, the incomprehensible sense of shock was accompanied by a complete lack of time and space to properly mourn my loss. Memories of my father's funeral remain vague and fragmented but I recall the absence of both my father's mother and siblings from the event – the result of a family rift emanating from simmering business tensions between my father and his brother. Any conversations within the

emotional realm were rare and the absence of adequate emotional comfort or support, akin to the British sense of keeping a 'stiff upper lip', pervaded family and school life. I recall the vast pile of condolence letters arriving in the ensuing weeks. As well as expressing sadness for the passing of my father they elicited references to my father's multiple sclerosis, of which I had no prior knowledge, and my sister who had died of a cot death some two years before I was born. Again, little was ever mentioned of her, and I felt I was hearing the news for the first time. As family secrets were coming to light, I struggled to make sense of them in the light of my father's death.

For two weeks after the funeral I remained at home contending with contradictory feelings of sadness and disbelief. I shed many tears during this time. Following my return to boarding school, I felt as if a tap had been turned off and the tears remained trapped inside for many years afterwards. It has only been within the past ten or fifteen years that I began to process the enormity of the experience.

Developmentally, I feel the loss of my father curtailed my childhood years, meaning I had to grow up and take responsibility for my life. This affected my education, with no one to push or guide me forward, leading to poor exam results and no desire to continue further education. ... the early childhood relationships with – and between my parents – provided a huge challenge in coming to terms with the loss of my father, as well as my personal relationships in adulthood.[16]

The death of a father can often lead to a major downturn in family finances if he was the main or only wage-earner in the family. As the son, you may feel now that it is your responsibility to provide this leadership and security. When John's father died the family house had to be sold within six months of the funeral and his mother moved three or four times in quick succession after that. His mother turned to him for practical help and support such as helping with the removals and completing practical DIY jobs around the house. This was not entirely unwelcome and John readily took on the 'father and surrogate husband role'. The sense of duty and responsibility helped him to feel identified with his father and also helped to bolster his feelings of low self-esteem and self-worth.[17]

The kinds of responsibility you may be expected to take on after the death of a parent are likely to be different after a mother or father dies. For boys, the death of a father can often lead to pressure to grow up and look after other members of their family, including their remaining parent. Winston's Wish therapists told Caspar Williams about the eulogy they'd heard read out by a headmaster from the school attended by two bereaved brothers, in which the headmaster emphasized 'how well they were looking after their mum'.

> Messages such as: 'well done for looking after your brother', or for 'being strong' or 'being brave', reward the child who does not appear to be overtly upset or breaking down. The need to contain one's emotions and keep grief locked inside can lead to heart-rending conclusions. … one young man coped with his grief quietly away from the rest of the family: "He waits until he goes to bed and then he has a cry under the covers."'.[18]

Paradoxically, even if your mother or father was not a great parent to you when they were alive, you may still miss an idealized version of them after he or she has died. A mother who was neglectful, critical and unsupportive while she was alive may, by dying, rouse great longings for the very characteristics she failed to embody. Similarly the death of an aggressive or a distant father can make you crave still more the father of your dreams who would nurture and protect you. It is as if by dying your mother or father has taken away forever the possibility of ever having those things. However strange it sounds, you can miss both the things your parent was and the things he or she failed to be. As Caspar Williams admits: 'Even if my father had survived, I do not believe that we would ever have had the type of relationship I yearned for.'[19]

Losing the same-sex parent

For children and teenagers, the death of a parent of the same sex as themselves is especially problematic. It causes a rupture in their developing identity that can be hard to mend, and many people speak of an inner emptiness that they have carried with them ever since their mother or father died.

Studies have found, for example, that girls bereaved of their mother are more likely to suffer from low self-esteem and anxiety later in life than either boys left with fathers, or boys or girls left with mothers.

Girls bereaved of mothers were also more badly affected than boys both in terms of school grades and anxiety, although boys who lost fathers were the group next worst affected.[20] Children aged between 6 and 12 are still forming their own sense of who they are in relation to their parents, and losing a same-sex parent at this stage is therefore very hard to cope with. The fact that they may still be too young to articulate or be fully conscious of the gender role their mother or father provided makes coping with their loss and distress all the harder. For these children, physical mementoes, such as photographs and belongings, as well as plenty of opportunities to talk about their dead parent, are essential.

The problems of arrested development, described earlier, are much greater when you are given little chance to 'update' your sense of who your parent was and what part they played in your life. Just as our understanding of living parents changes as we mature and develop, so our understanding of a dead parent should, ideally, change too. The difference is that, when a parent has died and is no longer there on a daily basis, other adults must play a much more active role in supplying information. Making space for children to talk and remember and reflect on their dead parent is a vital way in which their relationship with that parent can continue to keep pace with the child's own evolving sense of self.

It is not always easy to disentangle whether the difficulties girls experience are caused by losing a mother or by trying to relate to a grieving father. Probably, it is a mixture of both. Helen's mother died when Helen was 12. Her father could not bear to talk about his wife or to have reminders of her in the house. This made grieving for her dead mother very difficult and Helen grew up feeling as if some crucial part of her life had stopped at the moment when her mother died. Although now in her mid-twenties, she came for counselling because she was gripped by a sensation of being somehow 'unreal' and 'fake'. A turning point for Helen was discovering an aunt who not only was happy to talk about her dead sister, Helen's mother, but also had albums full of photographs that she was pleased to show her. Forming a relationship with her aunt gave Helen a bridge back to her own childhood, and slowly she was able to construct a sense of both who her mother had been and who she herself was in relation to her mother.

Teenagers are usually beginning to be able to see how their mother or father influences and informs their own sense of self. For this age group, the teenage son or daughter is right in the middle of working out how similar to and different from their same-sex parent they are, and their parent's death often throws this delicate and essential process into total disarray.

Even for grown-up children, the loss of a same-sex parent can be extremely hard, especially if there was ambivalence or conflict in the relationship. Judith, a teacher now in her mid-fifties, felt she had never been allowed to grow up in her mother's eyes. All her adult life she had struggled to prove her adult status to her mother by setting herself high standards in her working life and at home. She had always felt annoyed and constrained by her mother's view of her as somehow immature and childlike, but had also internalized that view to some extent. When her mother died, when Judith was in her late forties, she at first felt fantastically liberated. For the first time in her adult life she was released from the constraints of her mother's disapproval and from her own need to prove herself. But two years after her mother's death, Judith was extremely depressed, finding it hard to get up in the morning, not sleeping at night and feeling very anxious. Her mother's death had also removed Judith's sense of purpose and direction in life, leading to a real crisis in her sense of self.

> I was turning fifty, but I had no idea how to lead my life any more. All my adult life I'd taken my cue from my mother, from her idea of who I was, and now she was gone, I found I couldn't even get up in the morning. I'd got stuck at the age of about nine, which is how she saw me, and had never moved on from there. My adult life didn't really begin until my mother died.

A further, and deeply poignant, realization for Judith was that her mother had been 9 years old when her own mother had died in a car crash. The impact of her grandmother's tragically early death had made itself felt for at least two generations after. As Judith explains: 'Increasingly, I can see how my mother's bereavement as a child has affected not just the way she mothered me, but the way I've mothered my children too.'

When a girl's mother or a boy's father dies, it is not just the lack of a role model, but the lack of intimacy that is so hard to bear. You may miss the bedtime kiss your father always gave you before you went to sleep; or the game of football on a Saturday afternoon; or your mother's advice about clothes; or the regular phone call from her on a Sunday evening. Often people only become aware of this lost intimacy at key moments later in life. For me, getting married was a poignant occasion as it was my brother who walked me up the aisle in place of my father. Another woman, whose mother died when she was 8, was profoundly aware of the lack of female guidance throughout her teens and twenties:

> There was no one to tell me about periods, or teach me how to shave my legs, or put on nail varnish. When I had my first child, it hit me all over again: unlike the other women in the hospital, I had no mother to come and care for me and hold my newborn baby. My mother-in-law was wonderful, very loving and supportive, but I missed my own mother painfully.

One man, whose father died when he was in his teens, only realized much later in life how much he was affected by the complete lack of male role models in his family after his father's death. Now in his forties, he links his early childhood experiences and emotional deprivation – coupled with an inability to grieve for his father – to his depression and addictions in adulthood. His overeating provided a source of comfort and his difficulties in trusting people continues to be painful:

> I miss not having a father around to talk to for advice in times of need. When I hear men say I did this or that with my dad, I feel the loss of not being able to have that experience for many years. I realize now that I could have really benefited from a mentor in my adolescence and young parent years to help out in any which way a father could have. I regret that neither of my sons ever knew my father and vice versa.[21]

As Caspar Williams explains in his study of bereaved teenage boys, it is not simply the death of a same-sex parent that affects you, but the relationship you have with that parent before they died: 'While the loss of a father in adolescence certainly informed each co-researcher's sense of himself as a young man, his relationship with his father prior to death had an even greater impact on his male identity, or sense of being male.'[22]

Richard, another of the men interviewed by Williams, talked about his strong desire *not* to be like his father, and how this impacted upon his relationship with his own children and on his sense of self: 'The picture I grew up with of my father was a man who was a failure and who did not fulfil his potential.' He depicts his father as a man who was emotionally and physically detached from day-to-day family living while growing up; who lived off his inheritance and was a possible alcoholic.[23] The lack of a positive same-sex role model for Richard, combined with a sense of being alone and directionless in adulthood. Driven by the negative view of his father, Richard himself suffered, living his own life 'in rebellion against the image of that.'[24] Richard's experience highlights the enormous and sometimes highly destructive impact the surviving parent can have in terms of shaping your memories of a deceased parent. When asked how he had formulated this negative image of his father, Richard replied:

> It came from my mother. I remember many occasions, and even today I may hear words to the effect, [that] he wasted his life;

did not make use of his talents; he was lazy and a drunk. Yet (in hindsight) I do not recall receiving this message from the rest of his family, friends or even the men who worked for him on the farm.[25]

With the help of therapy and the Mankind Project, Richard was gradually able to take a more compassionate and balanced view of his father, which in turn helped him to be more forgiving and less judgmental towards himself:

It has taken me ages to accept [my father] was not a success in the world, but understanding that is not the whole person. I had a recent realisation when I was up in the North where my father had planted a lot of trees. I was standing in a field one day and, having managed this place for forty years, and knowing the kind of struggle it can be it just stood out: actually my father did OK![26]

All the men interviewed by Caspar Williams lamented the lack of opportunity to share a relationship with a significant male role model through adolescence into adulthood. They describe the absence of someone to rebel against whilst also trying to establish a sense of their identity within their peer group. Over-idealising their dead father was a problem for some, leading to a struggle to be a good-enough son or father, while for others, a negative view of the father could distort their sense of self and affect life decisions, such as career choice and marriage partner. Where the boy's early relationship with his father had been physically or emotionally distant, there were additional difficulties in discovering what exactly had been lost. As Williams explains:

The loss of the father deprives adolescent boys of an important male adult figure whom they can not only receive guidance from, but also rebel against. Without this, they often find themselves in an unboundaried existence where they are left to fend for themselves. ... [As a result] internalised defence strategies may occur, such as becoming fiercely independent or never asking for help. The death of the father severs an invisible bond of intimacy between father and son which never fully recovers, leading to impermanency in future relationships fuelled by a fear of further loss.[27]

On their residential weekends for bereaved children, Winston's Wish makes a point of having male volunteers in each group for just this reason. They recognize the important role that adult men play in modelling difficult emotions for the bereaved boys in the groups. For an adult male to demonstrate that it is all right to show his emotions, while retaining his masculine identity, is a huge relief to many of these boys, and may often be the first time they have ever seen men expressing emotions in this way.[28]

If the gender of the dead parent is an important factor in how you cope with their death, whether you are male or female seems to matter even more so. While bereaved boys show higher rates of overall psychological difficulties, with more aggressive and acting-out behaviour than bereaved girls,[29] girls exhibit more internalising symptoms, and are more likely to become severely depressed.[30] It's not that girls and boys don't both suffer, but they seem to react and cope differently to the pain and shock of losing a parent. The Joseph Rowntree Foundation interviewed 1,000 British teenagers at the age of 15 and then again at the age of 18, and found that 'for women, the death of a parent appears to have a markedly negative impact'. Forty-seven per cent of the girls who had experienced the death of a parent reported using drugs, compared with 20 per cent of those living with both parents. Forty per cent of bereaved girls had become pregnant by the time they were 18, compared with only 6 per cent of girls with two living parents.[31] Girls also have higher and longer-lasting rates of depression and anxiety after a parent's death than do boys. Initial levels of depression were not much different in girls and boys, but increased over time in girls, while they declined in the majority of boys, and researchers found a similar pattern with anxiety.[32] Three to four years after a parent's death, problems with depression and anxiety had usually decreased in boys, while for girls they were the same.[33] Furthermore these problems often didn't emerge until two years *after* their parent's death.[34]

Bereaved daughters are more likely than bereaved sons to act out their feelings in self-punishing behaviour, for example by eating too much or too little, or by repeatedly getting into destructive relationships. They may also set themselves very high standards at school and at home as if to compensate for the sense of failure that is often induced by a parent's death. One 14-year-old girl who came for counselling two years after her father's death had become obssessive about school work, studying far harder than was necessary for tests and exams. Although she vaguely understood that her compulsion to excel academically was a way of constructing order and structure in place of the emotional chaos and turmoil that she was really feeling, she was not able to act on this understanding and change her behaviour. By the time she was 16, her need to control her outer world was affecting her eating habits as well and she was regularly binging and vomiting to control her weight. It was at this stage that she realized that the grief she was still trying to avoid was in fact overwhelming her life, and she decided to seek help.

Girls (and women more generally) are more likely to experience persistent, negative thoughts after major stressful events than boys and men. Depressed feelings and anxiety are common reactions in boys and girls after a parent's death, but in boys they tend to fade steadily with time. The Family Bereavement Project, for example, found that girls were significantly more likely than boys to be suffering from prolonged grief and intrusive thoughts about their parent's death, *irrespective of age*. The girls reported more symptoms of persistent grief and a higher prevalence of prolonged grief disorder than boys. They were more likely to be struggling with strong bad feelings about the death, to be having trouble doing things they liked because of thinking how much better things were before the death, and to think about the death even when they didn't want to. Although for both boys and girls grief tended to decline over time, both normal and problematic grief decreased significantly more slowly in girls than boys. Six to nine years after the parent's death, significantly more girls than boys met the criteria for Prolonged Grief Diagnosis.[35]

Bereaved girls are more likely than boys to dwell on their feelings of unhappiness and loss, to focus passively on how bad they are feeling, and to draw negative conclusions about how they're feeling, for example, thinking they will never feel better. By contrast, teenage boys and men are more inclined to focus on problem-solving or distracting themselves.[36] Recent studies show that girls of all ages are more inclined to negative thinking than boys when they are asked to appraise the causes and consequences of their parent's death, and explain what it means for them. This way of thinking is in turn linked to depression and anxiety, so it creates a vicious circle.[37]

Bereaved girls, it seems, are more sensitive to and more harmed by threats to their interpersonal relationships, and are more reliant than boys on good personal relationships for well-being and recovery after a major bereavement. A parent's death doesn't create these problems, it simply highlights existing differences. Teenage girls, in particular, have an increased need for good, secure attachments as they move towards adulthood, and they are therefore more vulnerable in some ways when these attachments are ruptured or precarious.[38] This is also the stage of life when we first start to experiment with intimate relationships, and for teenage girls in particular their relationship with their fathers is very important to the development of their identity. This may be why teenage girls are particularly likely to run into problems after the death of a parent of either sex.

But it would be very wrong to draw the conclusion that boys are not also vulnerable after a parent's death. Indeed it may be that boys' coping strategies can shore up different kinds of long-term problems in adjusting to a parent's death. A study of 88 healthy adults, half of whom had experienced parental loss during childhood, found that those who'd lost parents had higher base rates of the stress hormone, cortisol, in their saliva than those who had no history of parental loss, and increased levels of cortisol in response to stress. This raised cortisol response was particularly so for men.[39] This seems to suggest that the loss of a parent in childhood is just as stressful for boys, but that stress shows itself differently. A 2006 study in America found that childhood parental loss was a *more* potent predictor of risk factors for depressive episodes in men than women.[40]

In general, men and boys are less likely to confide in others about what has happened to them and what they are feeling, and they are under more pressure from others and from society not to cry or break down or display symptoms of pain or vulnerability. Among teenagers, for example, boys tend to submerge their grief, with all its attendant emotions, hiding it away from themselves and others, often trying to block out painful thoughts and feelings with the help of alcohol, drugs and sex. This may make for particular problems for sons whose parents die since it is even harder for them to find support or recognition than it is for daughters, and these problems may not become apparent until much later in life. I have met men in their thirties, forties, fifties and even sixties who are for the first time emerging from decades of suppressed grief over a parent's death, who are only years later confronting their feelings of distress and loneliness, anger and confusion. A recent British study found that men who'd lost a parent during childhood were less likely to marry than either women bereaved in childhood or men and women whose parents had divorced. While women who'd been bereaved in childhood were more likely to be depressed in adulthood than any other group in the study, men were more likely to have avoided close relationships altogether.[41]

As Caspar Williams' research also shows, boys can appear to cope well in the short to medium term, with the deeper impact of a parent's death only emerging many years later. One was 13 when his father died. Now in his forties, he feels that his ability to grieve his father was continually overshadowed by the dramatic nature of the car accident which claimed his father's life and the 'continual dreams and fantasies' that his father would return and that life would resume much as before.

He and his father were in the new family van when his father lost control of the vehicle which tumbled over the edge of a nearby ravine. He recalls:

> I must have been thrown through the windscreen and thrown clear of it. I remember I was conscious and I had sustained some cuts to my face but otherwise I was okay. I remember scrambling up the slope and raising the alarm at home and my father was trapped in the car and the ambulance came and freed him and he was taken off to hospital ... I never dreamed for a moment that my father was going to die. I was mostly upset because we seemed to have lost his car which I had been so excited about.

It was only many years later, while explaining the circumstances surrounding the death of his father to his wife and children, that he was overwhelmed by strange emotions of loss and guilt for the first real time.[42]

Caspar Williams himself found that after the funeral was over, he suppressed most of his feelings about his father and about his death, and it wasn't until several decades later when he attended a Mankind Weekend that he was finally able to fully express his grief for his father's death.

> In the company of men and a strong facilitator, I was able to unlock the inner casket of my grief – enveloped within the deepest folds of the lower abdomen. Grief erupted, volcano-like, in waves of uncontrollable tears and emotion. I felt I was able to touch, feel and express the hidden love, sadness and anger that had been hidden away many years previously. I found a compassion and sense of understanding that I had never experienced within the male realm.[43]

Prolonged and delayed grief is not inevitable, however. Through a range of therapeutic interventions over a six-year period, the Family Bereavement Program succeeded in reducing complicated grief responses. Boys, interestingly, were most helped by the program, particularly in relation to problems with social withdrawal and detachment and insecurity.[44] Positive Psychology, Mindfulness, Emotional Intelligence and Cognitive Behavioural Therapy have also developed ways of helping people to manage thoughts and feelings after highly stressful life events and have been shown to be very effective in reducing anxiety and depression and strongly suggest that learning more about how our minds affect our emotions can be immensely helpful in reducing the risk of prolonged and complicated grieving in both children and adults.

Losing the living parent

On top of losing the parent who dies, one of the biggest changes you may have to face is the change that takes place in the remaining parent. Often you may feel you have lost not only the dead parent but the living one as well. This can happen in various ways and for various reasons: (i) because of the surviving parent's own grief; (ii) because he or she had not taken much of the load of parenting before and this now becomes obvious to you; (iii) because he or she remarries and becomes involved in a new life with a new partner from which you feel excluded.

For children and teenagers, how your relationship with your remaining parent develops after a death plays an important part in how well and how quickly you recover that trust. The more secure you feel in your relationship with your living parent, the more able you are to endure the pain of losing your other parent. The reason adults tend to cope better with the death of a parent than children or teenagers is because the remaining parent is far less likely to be the main source of support in their life. They will usually have a network of adult friends to turn to for support, and often a spouse or partner of their own. How your remaining parent grieves for their spouse will still affect you very deeply, but it is seldom central to how you construct the world and your place in it.

Coping with a parent's grief

Sometimes the remaining parent is so changed by grief that the person you knew seems gone forever. There may be profound physical change, such as loss or gain of weight, or loss of interest in appearance. This can be extremely distressing to witness. A formerly elegant mother can suddenly become a bedraggled, defeated old woman. A father who was a pillar of respectability can sit in front of the TV all day. It is not at all uncommon for parents to revert to adolescent or even childish behaviour after a bereavement, becoming irritable, unreliable, sullen and remote.

Julian hated watching his father grieving after his mother's death. He needed his father to be strong and reassuring and reliable. Instead he watched in dismay as his father turned into an overgrown teenager – slumped in front of the television, living on takeaways, filling the house with empty cans. 'He never drank beer at home before, let alone from cans,' Julian said, genuinely appalled by the change in his father. 'I had to go round picking them up, nagging him to turn the TV off.'

Even when the change is not so dramatic outwardly, you may sense an inner change that is equally alarming and distressing. To see parents vulnerable, hurt and helpless is very frightening, particularly if you have never before had cause to question their solid dependability, their emotional strength and their control over the world, yours in particular. You may have had plenty of cause to criticize them, you may have fought against their attitudes, values, opinions, politics and sexual morality; nevertheless they were still unquestionably there for you when you wanted them.

Seeing, or becoming aware, of your mother or father as an individual like yourself, capable of fear, sorrow, pain, and no more able to control the world than you, can shake your entire sense of the way things are. It is like being thrown to the ground by a second earthquake only moments after the first has devastated everything about you. Not only have you lost one parent, you now find you have lost two: the remaining parent is not the person you knew before. He or she may seem self-absorbed, not available for you to run to, unable to understand your feelings, perhaps not even *interested* in your feelings. You may find that suddenly *you* are the parent, the one taking responsibility for meals, bills, other siblings, while your so-called parent is like another child about the place: hopeless, helpless, dependent.

After my stepfather died my mother became very dependent on me for a while. Normally an independent, determined and capable woman, who got her children out of bed several hours earlier than we thought civilized, packed us off to music courses and activity weekends, organized us from one minute to the next, she was now suddenly transformed into someone who simply sat and stared and wept. I had to help her choose what clothes to wear, encourage her to eat, be a shoulder for her to cry on. She would come to me for help with the most straightforward tasks. It appalled me. I hated her being dependent on me. It made it difficult for me to grieve when I was so taken up with caring for her. There was no room or time for my own sorrow. Partly that was a relief: looking after my mother became a convenient excuse to avoid my own painful feelings, but it was also a great strain. I wrote in my diary at that time:

> Mum is like a child, unaware, incapable of nearly everything and always needing care and support and encouragement. The sight of her so weak and vulnerable frightens me, makes me back off emotionally. She often says how glad she is that we are close, that I am the only one who can understand how she feels, but I don't feel close at all. I hate her dependency. I find it revolting. I can't talk to her. I don't want her emotion. But I feel guilty

because I should be helping her if I can. I can't talk to her any-more. There is no one in the world for me to talk to now. I can't go to her and tell her how desperate I feel. She is the most dear person in the world to me and I try not to shut her up or out, but her needing me frightens me so much.

I was totally unprepared for my mother's frailty and weakness. I had no place for it in my idea of her. She was strong, independent, unflappable – or had been. Now that she was none of these things, I felt I barely knew her. My father had died, my stepfather had died, now it seemed I had lost my mother too.

As the weeks and months passed, she recovered her drive and deter-mination. It was a tremendous relief to me when, a couple of months later, I was able to write:

There are children playing a ball-game outside my window, shrieking with delight every time the ball goes bouncing into the mint patch, sending up a delicious waft of minty air. But best of all, I can hear Mum being efficient and competent downstairs in the kitchen, organizing the washing-up, goading Ellen into play-ing her violin. It is such a relief to be able to treat Mum like a person again.

What I really meant was that it was a relief to treat her like a *mother* again. Despite her recovery I still felt that our relationship had changed and that there was a new distance between us. I was wary of her possible demands and held her at arm's length. I also did not feel able to go to her with my problems, aware that she had so many of her own. I was often intolerant and unkind to her, perhaps to punish her for no longer being there for me, and although at times I felt overcome with remorse for being so impatient, for not being more understanding of what she was going through, I never felt those things quite strongly enough to stop myself. Somewhere inside I was horrified and furious that she was preventing me from being dependent, needy, scared and weak, by being those very things herself. As a parent, I thought, she was not supposed to be those things. Everything was topsy-turvy, all skew-whiff, all wrong.

Even after my mother had recovered her equanimity, I found it hard to overcome this feeling of having lost her too when my father and step-father died. I had seen her as a fallible human being, and with that insight came a new relationship, perhaps a more equal one in some ways, but not one which usually exists at this stage between a child and a mother.

In some ways, I had lost my mother as surely as I had lost my father and stepfather. I could never have back the all-supportive, all-encircling, all-protective mother of my childhood – a mother who was in any case more fantasy than past reality – and I grieved for that loss too. I did not want to be hauled into an adult world with adult perceptions and cold adult drafts howling around my ears. I did not want to know about death, or the weakness of the flesh, or the tiny frail thread that binds us to life, or how suddenly a heart can stop beating. I did not want to know about choice, and responsibility for myself, and powerlessness. Wasn't there anywhere to be a child still? The answer I gradually had to accept was: no.

Reassessing the living parent

Sometimes after one parent dies, you can realize that you had *already* lost the surviving parent. The parent who has died was actually the one doing *all* the parenting for you. At the very time of your greatest need, death has shone a harsh and unyielding light on the fact that the remaining parent had never really been there for you.

Charlotte was 23 when her father died suddenly of a heart attack. A year after his death, Charlotte was depressed, work was going badly and she was often taking days off and staying at home in bed. She avoided company except for very close friends. She could see nothing worthwhile in her life, nor any room for improvement. She thought her depression, and her other problems, might be connected with her father's death, but knowing this was no comfort, because his death was the worst of it all. The problem was not only accepting her father's death, but also having to face up to the parent her mother was not.

Charlotte adored her father and he adored her. He was all-important in her life. Her confidence and encouragement and love came from him. He praised her, encouraged her, advised her, supported her, made her feel worthwhile and important. He made her feel like a significant being in the world. Her mother, by contrast, had always been critical, hostile towards Charlotte's friends, jealous of Charlotte's relationship with her father, ungenerous emotionally, and psychologically unsupportive. After her husband's death, she relied heavily on Charlotte, but was no nicer to her. If anything she became even more carping and critical than before.

Nevertheless Charlotte felt responsible for her mother now that her father was dead. At a time when she needed to protect herself from criticism, to be with people who would be nurturing and gentle with her, she in fact spent more and more time with her mother, who profoundly and persistently undermined her confidence and exaggerated her feelings of

worthlessness and uselessness. Spending time with her mother only intensified her longing for her father; the painful presence of the former only
spotlighted the painful absence of the latter, aggravating her sense of
having lost her friend, comforter, supporter, encourager.

All her mother's criticism confirmed a picture of herself as 'bad' that
Charlotte had held inside from early childhood. Until her father's death,
his 'good' image of her and her mother's 'bad' image had battled it out,
and her father's had won. Now Charlotte had to fight for herself but,
grief-stricken, was in no fit state to fight. Instead she tried to make friends
with the enemy, unable to realize and accept that there was no real possibility for friendship there. The continual blame she received whenever
she saw or spoke with her mother after her father's death was especially
wounding when she herself was unarmed and vulnerable. To accept that
her mother could in no way make up for her father's absence was intol-
erably upsetting. Not only was Charlotte having to recognize the enormous importance of her father in her life and her vast need for him, she
was also having to recognize how destructive her mother was, and what a
negative influence she had always been.

For people who are older when a parent dies, who by then have their
own families and their own lives, there will have been time to recognize
and adjust to these realizations, to see the fallibility of your parents, to
seem them as people not just parents. With time most people come to
accept the shortcomings of their parents. If they are lucky they also come
to see their parents' achievements more clearly too. But there is a proper
time and place for these changes and just when one of them has died is
not the ideal time for a major reappraisal of your remaining parent. And
how are you to find the energy and emotional reserves to deal with these
issues when you are already drained by the effort of making some sense of
death itself?

For many people, as for Charlotte, the death of one parent is not only
dreadful in itself, but can often turn out to be the tip of an iceberg of loss.

Sometimes, however, the realization that you have an unsatisfactory or
non-existent relationship with the remaining parent can prompt more
positive changes.

Kate was also forced to reappraise her relationship with the remaining
parent, but for her the outcome was much happier. Her mother died
when she was 21 and she quickly realized just how little she knew her
father and just how little he had done as a father. 'He was the kind of
father,' she says, 'who'd come in from work, pat his children on the head
on the way through the living room, and disappear into his study for the
rest of the evening. We didn't know him at all. We never saw him. He
never spoke to us.' When her father took to saying to Kate and her sisters,

'You wish it had been me, don't you?' they knew there was some truth in his words. But six years on Kate can say unequivocally that she is glad her father did not die, because her mother's death forced them to get to know each other. 'I would never have known him otherwise, and now we have a real relationship and I'm very glad about that.'

But their relationship is not a traditional daughter-father one: Kate is not unusual in finding that, in a curious way, her father stopped being a parent in the way he had been before his wife died. Instead he became something closer to a friend or sibling. One immediate and significant change was that Kate's father stopped referring to his wife as 'Mummy' and began to use her Christian name. He also began to talk about Kate's mother as a person; someone he had loved and lived and argued with. His elevated role of parent, of father, vanished when the partner in his double act died. 'Dad started to talk about her in a way he never had before,' Kate recalls. 'He was much more open about their relationship, talked to us as if we were friends not daughters. At first I felt uneasy about it and resented that he wasn't doing more to look after us, but I've accepted it now.'

This kind of change is not so surprising when you consider that your parents may have presented themselves to you as parents, but to each other they were still two people who had once fallen in love and chosen to spend their lives together for better or worse. After one of them dies, it is that role that seems most significant to the remaining partner: the role of companion, supporter, partner and lover. A grieving father becomes first and foremost a grieving man; similarly a grieving mother becomes a woman who has lost her partner.

Losing a parent through marriage

A third way in which the death of one parent can lead to the loss of the remaining parent is through remarriage. Whether this happens six months after the funeral or three years after, it can be far more difficult to cope with than other people suppose. But it is certainly not uncommon for the remaining parent to remarry, particularly not for men, who are statistically far more likely to remarry than women. It is also not uncommon for people to remarry within a relatively short space of time: in an Australian study of 126 widows and widowers, all those who remarried did so within twelve to eighteen months of their spouse's death. Other studies have found that 60 per cent of widowers will remarry within two years of their first wife's death.

There are many reasons why men are more likely to remarry than women, emotional and sexual intimacy as well as for pragmatic reasons. If the marriage was organized along very traditional lines, many men will be unused to looking after themselves and their children on a day-to-day basis, feel overwhelmed by the business of washing clothes, shopping and cooking. Fathers are – still – often unable to cope with their children's needs and may welcome a woman to help with them. In *Facing Grief* Susan Wallbank suggests that there may be a connection between the high incidence of men remarrying and the fact that society discourages men from showing their emotions. This makes them far less likely than women to share their sorrow and their worries with friends, and more likely to form close attachments to new partners who can empathize and sympathize with what they are going through. In many cases men not only rely on women to share their feelings, but actually let women have the emotions for them. After the death of a partner, the need for emotional and physical closeness can be very great and it is certainly harder in Western society for men to find that solace from friends and relatives than it is for women to do so.

Whatever the reasons and whatever the timing, remarriage can be surprisingly hard to cope with. It may leave you with an acute sense of betrayal, may seem to deny the existence of the parent who died, may seem to reduce him or her to total insignificance.

You may well feel considerable anger towards your remarrying parent. There seem to be so many unacceptable thoughts: 'It's all right for Mum to have someone to comfort her, but what about someone to comfort me?' There is the voice that says, 'So how much did Dad really love Mum if he has found someone new so soon?' There is the awful feeling that your dead parent is going to be replaced somehow, and nagging concerns that you will be expected to love this person, call them Mum or Dad, or have to be told what to do by this stranger in your home. You may well draw comparisons between the new partner and your dead parent. You may feel that the parent you had relied on for love and support has abandoned you, has withdrawn, wrapped up in this new relationship with no time or feeling or concern left over for you. Even if you were close, it can feel as if a wall has sprung up between you and your parent. They are always busy, never there when you need them, your requirements have to take second place because of the new person in their life.

On top of the hurtfulness of all that, there is often a sense of disgust, repugnance: 'How could they? How could they be happy again, so soon?' Realizing that parents can be weak, fearful and vulnerable, often feels like an additional loss, and in the same way so can realizing that they are sexual beings who need physical affection, feel desire and are desirable. In Shakespeare's play, *Hamlet,* the revulsion and betrayal which a child can feel when one parent dies and the other embarks on a new sexual relationship are powerfully evoked. Hamlet rages about his mother:

> ... within a month,
> Ere yet the salt of most unrighteous tears
> Had left the flushing in her galled eyes,
> She married. O! most wicked speed ...

He makes the common mistake of the young in thinking older people incapable of sexual desire. 'You cannot call it love,' he says to her, 'for at your age the hey-day in the blood is tame.' He is disgusted, enraged and bewildered by the fact that she is now not only a mother to him, but a woman acting on her own needs and desires as a sexual being. Hamlet is an extreme case, perhaps, but many of these feelings are there in lesser forms when a parent remarries.

Within a year of his father's death when he was a teenager, John's mother started a new relationship. John recalls feeling incredibly angry with his mother who had degenerated into a 'lovesick teenager', as he puts it, in relation to her new partner. 'She would write down daft poems.'[45] When my mother remarried after eight years of widowhood, I oohed and aahed sincerely enough at the photographs of her wedding day, but I could not quite cope with the one of her and her new husband kissing on the mouth. In fact I found the whole business of my mother being in love pretty hard to handle. At her age! I recently met a man in his fifties whose widowed father had started a new relationship. 'My mother's only died a year ago,' he said. 'Dad wants me to meet this new woman, but I don't want. It's far too soon.' What he meant was that it was far too soon *for him*.

There is no doubt that having to negotiate a network of new relationships on top of the strain of a major and often recent bereavement is a daunting task for many grieving children. Yet surprisingly little is known about the child's experiences of growing up in a stepfamily. Two assumptions conspire to keep it that way: the first is that stepfamilies are the product of divorce, not death; the second is that remarriage following a husband's or wife's death is a sign of recovery and therefore 'a good thing'. Neither of these is necessarily true. The stereotypical figure of the wicked stepmother is familiar enough from stories like Cinderella, Snow White and Hansel and Gretel, as is the ineffectual father who usually lurks in her shadow. Both have some grounding in real life. A recent study found that two-thirds of stepchildren actively disliked their stepmothers. Far from being a supportive presence, many stepmothers in this study were strict, critical and intolerant of their stepchildren. In addition, they often stood in the way of the child's relationship with the father. One woman remembers how her father used to apologize for not being nicer, but said that his new wife 'doesn't like me talking to you'.[46] At a time when this girl needed emotional closeness from her remaining parent, her need was doubly frustrated, first by death and then by her father's remarriage.

When a widowed mother remarries the reverberations are not quite so extreme. But it depends very much on the stepfather. Some take a side-line from the start and are careful to stay there, not intervening in any significant way; others are keen to take charge and assert their authority. Added to the sense of being displaced from the centre of the remaining parent's life, this can be a very painful change for many bereaved children. A 15-year-old boy who came for counselling four years after his father's death because of problems at school quickly disclosed the real source of his anxieties: his mother was on the verge of remarrying a man whom Tom disliked and distrusted. Since his father's death, Tom had taken a very protective role towards his mother and they had developed a close and confiding relationship. This had changed since his mother had met her boyfriend, and Tom was now feeling marginalized and rejected without quite realizing it. In addition, his stepfather-to-be had moved in while Tom was at boarding school on the other side of the country and, when Tom had gone home for the holidays, he'd found him very much at home there, even ticking Tom off for breaking some minor house rules, such as wearing his shoes indoors. In part his mistrust and unhappiness was a reaction to the clumsy way in which his mother and her future husband were handling their relationship, but his sense of dislocation was also related to the way he had responded to his father's death four years earlier. Keen not to overburden his grieving mother with his own pain, he had pushed his feelings of grief out of sight and thrown himself into the role of little protector to his mother. With his mother no longer needing him in this way, there was some space for Tom's own grief to emerge at last. This was very frightening for Tom, who was now left feeling unprotected himself, angry with his mother for abandoning him and angry with his mother's boyfriend for 'taking her away' from him. Tom was struggling with these intense and complicated emotions without any obvious adult support: his teachers at school were oblivious to the domestic upheavals in his home life, many of them were not even aware that his father was dead, and back home his extended family were all in favour of his mother's impending marriage, relieved that she was no longer going to be 'on her own'. No one had given much thought to how Tom was feeling or coping.

When the surviving parent remarries, their life appears to be moving on, while for the children it may feel as if a major hammer blow has just landed on their heads. The loss of closeness with your living parent is like a rerun of your earlier loss, and the fear and uncertainty about what the future in this new family unit holds is also uncomfortably reminiscent of the anxieties that crowded in after your parent's death.

After her mother died of cancer, Sue experienced all three ways of losing a living parent: she felt she lost her father first of all through his grief, then through her own reappraisal of their relationship, and finally through his remarriage.

Sue's mother died when she was 18 and within a few months Sue's father fell in love with a friend of the family and decided to remarry. The woman was also widowed and had two children by her previous marriage. Not only did Sue have a 'new mother' to cope with – and of course this 'new' father – she also had a new set of siblings. In the next couple of years Sue became moody and easily disheartened when things went wrong. She left university, started to do a design course but dropped out after a week, decided to travel round the world, but somehow ended up working as a secretary for a local firm and living at home. She also started to have a series of relationships, all of which began very intensely and ended very rapidly. Furthermore, all her relationships seemed to happen simultaneously, as if she were incapable of committing herself to any one person at any one time. Sue did not at all enjoy the complications and deception this habitual two-timing involved, but she found it impossible to break the pattern.

It was as if she herself were split in two: there was the part of herself that was pleased for her father and the part that was angry and disappointed with him. There was the part of her that liked her stepmother and the part that hated her for usurping her mother. She partly liked having a new brother and sister, but partly hated the intrusion of these strangers into her life. There was the part of her that also wanted, like her father, to be able to forget the pain of her mother's death and fall in love and be healed, but there was a part of her that wanted to keep her mother alive by not entering into life and love again. She was divided within herself, by split loyalties to her father and to her mother, and by split ideas about how life should proceed after her mother's death.

Distracted and vague at the best of times, Sue's father was even more so now, in the throes of both grief and new love. Not by any means an unkind man, he simply did not notice what his daughter was up to, and if he did, he put it down to her age and the death of his wife. Sue's predicament was like that of the man in Stevie Smith's poem, 'Not waving but drowning':

> Nobody heard him, the dead man,
> But still he lay moaning: I was much further out than you thought
> And not waving but drowning.

Sue lost her father through remarriage and she lost him because he was not there in her life as she needed him to be. It was several years before she accepted that he could never replace her mother in the sense of being an active, guiding presence. But until she began to accept that, she was trapped by her anger with him for having 'disappeared' when she so needed him, and trapped into self-destructive behaviour by her need both for support and revenge.

How your remaining parent behaves and reacts is extremely important in how you yourself adjust to the death of your mother or father. The younger you are when a parent dies, the more this is so. Your remaining parent – assuming you have one – is a vital combination of lifeline and role model. They provide you with a link to your dead parent and also with an example of how to grieve for them.

Hope Edelman has described how terrified she was that her father would collapse completely after her mother's death, and how she and her other siblings made it difficult for him to express his grief, but also how they took their cue from his lack of emotion and tried not to express theirs. After my stepfather's death, I had the opposite problem: I was appalled by my mother's open and distressing displays of grief. I hated witnessing her vulnerability and I hated my inability to make things better. Her grieving so easily – as it seemed to me – only made it harder for me to work out what I was feeling. I reacted by retreating into myself, wary of placing any more pressure on my clearly overwhelmed mother, fearful of being the cause of her total collapse.

In *Motherless Daughters*, Edelman outlines four types of unsupportive father that a bereaved child may find herself having to deal with and her categories apply just as readily to children who are left with a grieving mother.

First of all there is the 'I'M OK, YOU'RE OK PARENT'. This is the parent who locks up the true pain of grieving behind a determined facade of coping. They exert considerable pressure, often without intending any harm, on everyone in the family to conceal their grief from each other, themselves and the outside world. All their energy is diverted away from what they are really feeling into adjusting and coping on a practical level. Clothes are thrown out, possessions are given away, rooms are rearranged with great efficiency, but little time or care is taken over the feelings associated with these changes. This kind of parent is perhaps the most dangerous, because he or she leaves so little space for genuine emotion. The dead parent and the past they represent is set firmly – but inappropriately – aside.

The second type of parent is 'THE HELPLESS PARENT', who allows feelings of grief to overwhelm him or her. This is the mother or father who leans heavily on the children for emotional and practical support, without proper concern for how burdensome this can feel, nor for the long-term damage it can cause to a child's emerging sense of self, who must suddenly become a pseudo-spouse, or even a parent to the parent. The child's natural desire to be protected by a parent becomes confused with the desire and the need to do the protecting. Children with this kind of remaining parent often become 'old before their time' and later experience feelings of inauthenticity, sometimes 'breaking out' of their adult lives to take the years they missed out on first time round. Teenagers of parents who react to a partner's death in this way often have particular difficulties with their emerging sexual identities as a result of the confusion in family roles. There may be conscious or unconscious anxieties, for example, about the emotional intimacy between a mother and son, or father and daughter. The uneasiness that this kind of situation can produce in the teenaged child can make it extremely difficult for them to form intimate relationships with people of his or her own age: reminders of their emerging sexuality are strenuously avoided. On the other hand, I have also come across teenagers who have gone the other way, and become sexually hyperactive in an attempt to prove to themselves how normal they are, and thus combat their sense of discomfort about blurred boundaries and muddled roles with their remaining parent.

Next comes 'THE DISTANT PARENT', who is unable to sustain a connection to the parent who has died and who with time finds it increasingly difficult to maintain proper contact with his or her children. This is the father who remarries and quickly hands over the emotional and practical care of his children to his new wife, not realizing how impossible a task that is, nor how unsatisfactory from the children's point of view. This is the divorced mother who cannot sympathize with her children's grief for a person who caused her only unhappiness. This is the parent of either sex who manages to keep tending to the children's physical needs, but no longer has the energy or inclination to engage emotionally. This kind of parent inflicts a cruel double loss on a bereaved child, and can profoundly undermine his or her ability to trust and to love in the future. Sometimes the presence of another supportive and emotionally engaged adult can mitigate the effects of this kind of parental reaction. A 16-year-old boy, whose father had died and whose mother had withdrawn from him emotionally, found himself a 'second home', receiving from the parents of a school friend the stability, responsiveness and support he so urgently needed. While his relationship with his mother remained cool and restrained for many years, he drew great strength from his warm and loving relationship with his friend's parents, the mother in particular. At the age of 32, himself happily married with a 2-year-old son, he attributed his recovery from what was in effect a double bereavement to the love he'd received from this second family.

Finally, there is 'THE HEROIC PARENT'. This is the mother or father who is so wrapped up in how well she or he is coping that they somehow overlook the less successful progress of their children. Like the 'I'm OK, you're OK parent', they effectively impose their emotions on to their offspring, not allowing room for different ways of grieving. This type of parent again puts a great deal of pressure on a bereaved son or daughter to 'keep up', to adapt to the remaining parent's version of how things are going, and as a result leaves little space for the child's own reaction to a parent's death. This is the parent who elicits congratulations and admiration from other people outside the family, but who exerts a disguised emotional tyranny. This is the mother who takes a full-time job so that the family won't have to move house and who after work rushes home to cook, clean and sort the laundry. This is the father who works full-time but makes sure he gets to his children's sports days and end-of-term concerts now that his wife can't. This is the parent who makes the grieving child feel so small and insignificant and yet so much trouble. These are the parents who really do try to do their best by their children and yet, by stretching themselves to their limits, can often end up burdening their children with a sense of responsibility. These are the children who in later life are likely either to set themselves punishingly high standards ('My mother managed, so why can't I?'), or else become directionless and unmotivated ('I can never do what Dad did; I'm bound to fail').

For younger people who lose parents, the remaining parent is not only a role model for grieving, he or she is also a lifeline between you and your dead parent. This is particularly important for children and teen-agers, who will not have a fully formed sense of their dead parent, in the way they might have done later in life. I know that my own grieving has been greatly complicated by the fact that I didn't know my father all that well. Despite being a tremendously important figure in my life, symboli-cally and actually, my father was nevertheless an enigma to me. This was partly because of circumstances: I hadn't lived with him since I was 5. And it was partly because, even years after their divorce, my mother couldn't bring herself to tell me anything other than how awful he'd been as a husband. Her view of him clearly didn't tally with mine and I gradually learnt to stop asking her about him. Both before and after his death, this made the business of knowing my father far from simple. As I got older, and my perspective changed, there were more not fewer questions in my mind about who he was.

When a parent dies, you are left with the difficult task of continuing a two-way relationship on your own. How you relate to your dead parent is determined partly by how old you are, not just when they die, but right through your life. How you think about your parent will change as you change. A child who was 6 when her mother died will understand both her mother and her death differently by the time she is 12, and will have changed again by the time she is 18 and 24. People whose sense of their dead parent does not evolve in this way are the ones who are likely still to feel damaged and haunted by their bereavements years and years later. They are 'stuck in the past' in the real sense of the expression.

The remaining parent is often the only person with whom you can talk, reflect, check. The extent to which he or she is able to respond to your continuing need for information and clarification about your dead parent will help or hinder you in the task of learning to live with your loss. Mary was in her mid-twenties when she finally told her mother to stop talking about 'Daddy'. As Mary explains, 'I was ten when my father died, and my mother talks about him as if I were still ten. But he's not "daddy" in my mind any more. I'm a grown up and I see him as a grown up, not as a child.'

When your own remaining parent cannot provide you with either the role model or the lifeline you need, try to find other adults who can be those things for you. I learnt with time that there were people I could talk to – my aunts, adult friends of the family, my grandmother and one of my siblings eventually gave me the opportunities I needed to get to know him a little better after his death than his short lifetime allowed me to do. Even if your living parent cannot help in this respect, finding someone in your life who can help you to fill the gaps in your knowledge about the parent who has died will help to buffer you to some extent from the double loss that many bereaved children experience, and help you to continue to build an ongoing relationship with them.

Losing the living parent is a lot to take on board at a time when the boat you are on already feels pretty shaky. You may find yourself feeling resentful or angry as a result, either towards your remaining parent or towards the one who has died. You may feel they have failed to look after you, failed to protect you from the harshness of the world; that by dying or remarrying, or simply by being grief-stricken themselves, they have let you down badly. You may hate your dead parent for dying and leaving the family with so many problems to sort out alone. You may hate the living parent for failing to sort out those problems. It takes time to understand how you are affected by these changes, and time to get used to the changes themselves.

Losing your faith

People generally assume that religious faith will help you through difficult times in your life, but you may in fact find that your religious faith is no help at all. On the contrary, you may feel that it is failing you just when you need it most, and that your parent's death makes a mockery of faith in God. You may ask yourself: how can there be a just God when this has happened? You may feel that your sorrow and pain proves there cannot be a caring God.

The sensation of having been let down by God and by your faith at the same time that so much else that was solid in your life seems to be collapsing can be the cause of great despair and anguish. It is as if there is nothing left to hang on to any more, no source of hope, no core of goodness. To lose your faith on top of everything can add considerably to your feelings of hopelessness and pointlessness. If your faith is important to you, it may be worth finding someone with whom you can discuss your feelings and doubts. One rabbi I spoke to about the additional stress caused by loss of faith after a parent's death suggested: 'If there is anger at God, tell him. Tell him that you feel cheated and let down. It is important to be angry.' But once you have done that, he said, you should take a look at your expectations of life and of God.

> Religion is there not to stop awful things happening, but to help you when they do happen. God is not a divine vending machine where you put in your coin and get out what you want. God is someone to turn to, to help you deal with life as it is, not to change it.

Different religions will have different approaches to the feelings of the bereaved. It is important to hang on to the fact that your feelings of anger have their place – religious faith worth having will make room for that anger, not deny it.

Losing your base

When things are changing fast in your life, you need a still point of reference, a place or situation that remains solid and dependable.

Unfortunately, it is precisely this still point of reference that is often missing after a parent's death.

My stepfather died while I was at university and I found it very difficult that the firm base of my home was not there for me. I went away each term and came back in the holidays to find the people and places I had left behind more changed than the one I had gone away to. I needed stability, but it was no longer to be found at home. Rooms were rearranged; furniture sold; books and possessions boxed up or thrown away. My mother was distracted, anxious, frantically overworked. My little brother and sister mothered her. It was all very strange and bewildering.

Other friends who were also trying to adjust after a bereavement were having the same difficulty: their need for a secure base to return to, in order to be with people who understood them, was frustrated, because 'home' was where most of the change was taking place.

Maria could not stand the feeling of being totally adrift. In her first term at university she was surrounded by new people and places. At home everything had changed radically since her mother's death. She so hated feeling that, while she was away, her home was disappearing altogether, that she decided to take a year off and go back home to be with her father and sister. At least there she could see what was changing, rather than being abruptly confronted with the changes when she came home in the holidays.

Carina, on the other hand, decided to go to college as planned. Her father had died very recently and the start of her first term coincided with the rest of her family deciding to move to another part of the country. She felt very isolated at college, so far from her family, but she was determined to stick it out. Years later she realized how hard it had been for her to have all these changes taking place simultaneously, but at the time Carina focused all her energy on the need to 'settle down' at college, make friends, fit in. She was often confused by how difficult she was finding it, but didn't relate these difficulties to all the huge changes in her life. For Carina, the easiest option was to make college the firm base, and that was what she worked to create.

Losing your memories

Even when you yourself have decided to throw things away, losing things can be hard. One of the reasons why it can be so distressing is because possessions are often intimately bound up with memories, and memories are precious and fragile to you now. There is often a real fear that once the clothes and books and records have been given away or you have left the home where you and your parent lived, you will no longer be able to remember your parent properly, that the death will somehow happen all over again in the failure of your memory.

When his father died, Alan sat in his bedroom and every single thing around him reminded him of his father. When a few years later his mother remarried and the house was reorganized to accommodate her new husband, Alan moved to a different room in the house. Dismantling his bedroom was excruciatingly painful, because in his mind it was so bound up with his father: these triggers of photographs, books and ornaments had helped keep his father alive for him.

If, for whatever reason, you are not able to keep belongings that mean a lot to you, then at least allow yourself to think about what the object really represents for you: does it remind you of your parent's sense of humour or some other lovable and particular characteristic? If you can focus on the specific value and significance of the object that is lost, you may well find that the memory of the cherished aspect of your mother or father is still with you.

As William Worden says, people bereaved in childhood and adolescence need to develop:

> an inner representation of the dead parent that allows him or her to maintain a relationship with the deceased, a relationship that changes as the child matures and the intensity of grief lessens. The child negotiates and renegotiates the meaning of the loss, and in time, relocates the dead person in his or her life and memorializes that person in a way that allows life to move on.[47]

Memories and possessions are a vital way in which we remember and memorialize a parent who has died.

I still have a jumper of my father's that has long been too full of holes actually to be worn, but I cannot quite bring myself to throw it away. Apart from the jumper and a photograph, I have few physical reminders of him. Over the years I have honed down the mementoes and memory joggers, the physical signs of my father, but I have done so very gradually, almost without noticing, letting go of things as I no longer feel the need for them; along with this has come, also gradually, a slowly increasing confidence that my father is alive in my memory, that he will not fade away to nothing. I know now, though no one could have told me this, that the memory is solid, unshakeable, sometimes more powerful, sometimes less so, but always there. I don't have access to memories of every single moment we ever spent together, but over the years the familiar memories come and go and I have found myself remembering new things too.

The only way my father could cease to be, would be if I died myself. The very fact that I exist reminds me of him. I am here because of him, my existence is proof of his existence, and a constant reminder of him – sometimes comfortingly, sometimes less so. As long as I live, so he lives in me, in my memories of him and in the part of me that is him. I have heard other people say this too. One woman expressed it perfectly when she said about her father's death: 'Only half of that relationship died, the part of it that was him. The other half, the half that is me, is still alive.'

Memories are a vital way of keeping someone alive. In parts of Africa, some tribal people do not regard eternity as something that exists in the future, instead they see eternity as stretching out *behind* them, and when they die they join, in their turn, the eternal beings who live forever in the flesh and in the memories of the living. Each new generation keeps alive the previous one through memory. Nomadic people attach great importance to the past. When you cannot locate yourself by a specific place, the sense of continuity must come through attention to who your ancestors were. You learn where you come from in terms of people rather than places: lineage becomes very important.

It is by using memory in this way that bereaved people keep the past alive. Phyllis Silverman and Steven Nickman have described this as becoming 'a living legacy'. This is not the same as trying to pretend the dead are not dead, but rather a gift that enables you to keep alive a meaningful and positive connection between you and loved ones who are dead.

Losing your youth

Perhaps the greatest and most traumatic loss after a parent's death is the loss of your youth. People of all ages may feel this, but for children and teenagers especially, the sense of having to 'grow up overnight' is one of the most common and often difficult aspects of bereavement. Responsibilities come suddenly and these external pressures can accentuate the inner feeling that your youth is over.

People often said to me after my father died, 'Well, at least you're young. Young people are more resilient.' How unhelpful and how hurtful I found that comment! Because the other side of being young when a parent dies is that you are not so ready for it, you have fewer resources for dealing with it, and you are less supported afterwards. Friends, however well-meaning, are often unable to help simply because they do not really know what you are going through. They do not know and cannot guess how long you go on feeling miserable and lost and directionless, how long you go on missing your parent. Relatives and friends of the family often make the same mistake, thinking that because you are young, you will 'get over it' quickly.

I was lucky in knowing a couple who had been close friends of my father. They did not try to sweep my feelings under the carpet. The husband had been through the death of his mother at the age of 14 and understood very well what I was going through. I often used to go and spend a couple of hours with them at weekends, and they were the only people who really just let me sit and be miserable and miss Dad without feeling ashamed of not having 'got over it by now'. I am still very grateful for their understanding and their help in keeping him alive in memory – not conspiring to kill his existence and importance to me through silence, as so many others do out of a combination of ignorance, insensitivity and embarrassment.

Before adolescence, assuming life has gone relatively smoothly, your faith in the world is still usually intact. Your trust in your parents as people you can rely on to be there, to care about you, is still unbroken and unquestioned. Their death at this stage of your life destroys that faith and trust. Children who lose a parent are often forced to see the world with a perspective beyond their years. A 6-year-old shows an awareness of other people's feelings inappropriate for so young a child. A 9-year-old must help with the housework far more than any of his friends. A 12-year-old looks after her younger siblings as if she were their mother.

The sense of inner confusion this creates for the child cannot be underestimated. In *Motherless Daughters,* Hope Edelman describes how she became the 'rock' of her family in the face of her father's inability to cope or endure the loss or grief. Seventeen at the time, she took over responsibility for her younger siblings, taking her brother for haircuts, her sister to the dentist, even inheriting her mother's car. 'I stepped on a fast forward button that transported me from seventeen to forty-two.' When she left home the following year to go to university, her 15-year-old sister took over these roles. But fast forwarding through a crucial stage of her development created real problems further down the track. She describes the sense of inner disjunction she experienced, the longing to reunite 'seventeen' and 'forty-two' into a coherent adult self, and the difficulty of doing so.

This sense of 'arrested development', of there being black holes in one's identity, is deeply undermining. It leaves you with a feeling of being somehow insubstantial and inauthentic. It is not at all uncommon for people who have lost a parent during their childhood or adolescence, when their personality is still developing, to get stuck, developmentally speaking, at the age they were when their parent died. This is one way in which children and young people protect themselves from the full impact of grief and loss. It is the emotional equivalent of the way in which memory blocks out visual recollections after extremely traumatic events, often for years and years afterwards.

Another way in which children defend themselves against grief is by displacing their own feelings onto someone or something else. The little girl who says, 'I wonder if mummy is lonely in heaven' is actually wondering how she will survive her own feelings of loneliness. Feelings of great neediness and longing can also be transferred onto another person, maybe a parent, a teacher, a friend or a sibling. When Princess Diana was killed in 1997 after her chauffeur-driven car spiralled out of control on a Paris underpass and crashed, her brother, Viscount Althorp, was clearly devastated. His intense reaction to his sister's death became more understandable when one learnt that their parents had divorced when they were very young and their mother had left them. Diana, in his own words, had become 'like a mother' to him. It is not improbable that as a small child, he had displaced his longing for his own mother onto his protective older sister, and that when Diana then died in sudden and tragic circumstances, he found himself grieving for the mother he'd lost so many years before as well as for his beloved sister. Princess Diana, too, bore the legacy of her mother's absence during her childhood, a legacy that found expression in her much-vaunted caring for others – again a textbook case of displaced and transferred need.

Children who lose parents when they are still young can carry with them into adulthood a residual fear of emotional involvement or commitment of any kind. They may be very independent, reluctant to trust others with their feelings. They may avoid emotional intimacy altogether, or they 'prove themselves right' by continually getting into destructive, hopeless relationships. They may on the other hand try to embody the things they feel they lost by becoming highly dependable, responsible, always there for others. Adults who lost parents when they were young often become overachievers, driving themselves to extraordinary limits, perhaps to compensate for an inner feeling of failure, or perhaps in response to a learnt pattern of self-denial. A study of famous men throughout history found that a significantly large proportion had lost their mothers in childhood or adolescence (Beethoven, Michelangelo, Darwin, Hegel, Abraham Lincoln to name but a few). And the same applies to women. Marie Curie, George Eliot, Virginia Woolf, Eleanor Roosevelt, Madonna – all lost mothers in early life. Virginia Woolf once said that she only became a writer because of her mother's death.

A parent's death when you are young leaves its mark one way or another. Death comes as more of an outrage, more of a shock than when you are older. Even at the age of 18, 20 or 24 you have barely admitted to yourself that death is real. You may have read books or seen films in which the hero dies and been moved by it; you may have written poems and stories about death; you may have lain in bed at night fantasizing about being orphaned and how terrible it would be. You may well have wished your parents dead on occasion. But it is still the *very last thing* you actually expect to happen. Death is not yet part of your experience nor part of the framework of your life.

What makes coping with death so hard at this age, and what other people often cannot comprehend, is that in some ways you are no longer like other young people. In my experience and the experience of others I have talked to and worked with, it is the sense of isolation that makes death particularly hard to cope with at this age. You may well feel isolated from everyone: family, relatives, friends. You are not part of an adult world – in their eyes or yours – yet you no longer belong as before with the younger world of your friends and contemporaries. I remember feeling very responsible for my friends, fearing for their lives as they set off down some country lane driving far too fast with far too much beer in their blood. They were excited, having fun; I was downright terrified. All I could think about was how dangerous it was, how they ought to be more careful, how awful it would be for their families if they were killed. I was always in the back seat saying: 'Could you slow down a bit … '. I felt a degree of responsibility for them that they certainly did not feel for themselves. I was fearful for their lives while they were careless. They still believed in their own immortality; I knew they were all too mortal. I wanted to be as happy-go-lucky, as carefree, as fast-living as they, but I couldn't be, however much I wanted to, because the world around me felt now an unsafe, risky place, and death all too real a possibility.

What you lose when a parent dies is this fragile but important illusion of immortality – yours no less than your parent's. Death shows you like nothing else just how fragile you are, just how insecure is your grasp of the mortal coil, how quickly and easily a life can end, and how totally final it is when that happens. The absoluteness of death is deeply shocking when it first affects your life. Nothing prepares you for it, and nothing reduces the shock of its impact. The world looks different because suddenly the world *is* different. Your view of the world is quite different. When someone you love dies at this stage of your life, you are left in a kind of limbo between youth and adulthood which can be a very lonely, frightening place. This sense of having lost your youth is something that also needs to be mourned.

7

CHANGES AND LOSSES
The public kind

One change leaves the way open for the introduction of others.

Machiavelli

The changes and losses described so far are ones that may well be painfully obvious to you without being very apparent to people beyond your immediate family. They are changes and losses that you have to cope with privately, with relatively little support. Other changes in your life, however, will be more noticeable to the outside world. Moving house, changing jobs, ending a relationship: these kinds of change are not specifically related to a bereavement and are not considered at all out of the ordinary. As changes, they will be generally recognized, but as *losses*, which for you they are also, the significance of these events may be entirely lost on other people. For this reason, these 'ordinary' changes and losses can be particularly hard to bear.

Losing your home

Moving house is always an upheaval and unfortunately a parent's death often makes such a move unavoidable. Moving house, however, is more than a time- and energy-consuming nuisance: it is an event that can arouse intensely painful feelings. If possessions are bound up with memories, how much more so are places.

In *The Trauma of Moving*, Audrey T. McCollum describes how, even at the best of times, moving can be upsetting. Her book is primarily a psychology textbook about the effects on women of moving, but her conclusions have a wider relevance. She quotes one of her interviewees as saying: 'Moving is like dying. I felt at one with my home. I was afraid of losing it, of feeling alone. It's like dying, because dying means aloneness.'

Summing up, McCollum states that:

> Moving [means] experiencing psychological homelessness ... an interruption of the sense of continuity, and a loss of feelings of mastery. This limbo kindles anxiety in the present and rekindle[s] anxiety from the past. ... Moving [means] enduring disorientation, confusion, disorganization – a loss of control, a temporary loss of the sense of competence that is a foundation of self-esteem.

When it comes on top of other losses, moving home can be particularly distressing. The relocation of your physical belongings and self means dislocation from where you were before. Unless you feel very secure and steady inside yourself, which is highly unlikely in the circumstances, that dislocation will probably be extremely painful. You are losing part of yourself, the part of you that lived in that home, the connection with things that happened while you lived there, and the connection with the people and possessions you lived there with. Places keep memories alive. Going back to a place invariably stirs memories and leaving a place invariably stirs them too. It stirs a sense of the past slipping away.

After a parent's death it is unfortunately often necessary to move house, whether because of shortage of money, or a need for the remaining parent to be closer to work, relatives or schools. But to lose your home and the familiarity of your surroundings at a time when everything feels so strange and fragile is hard. It can feel as if nothing is left untouched by this death. It is reaching out and spoiling every aspect of your life. The process of dismantling your home and packing up belongings can feel extremely destructive, especially at a time when so much in your life seems to be falling apart.

Understanding that packing and moving are *always* stressful and that when you are already sensitized to loss, separation and instability, they will be especially so, can help you accept and tolerate these uncomfortable feelings. Your reactions are not abnormal: to feel nothing at such a time would be far stranger.

Losing your job

When Michael left his job in a publishing company, a job he had never enjoyed, to set up in business as a furniture maker, he failed to realize that this change would involve loss. He expected to be relieved, liberated and full of zeal for his new life. Instead he became depressed, listless and lacking in confidence. Four years earlier his mother had died of multiple sclerosis and as his change of job came fairly soon after her death, he was less able to cope than he might have been. Even though it was a change he had chosen and wanted, it involved substantial loss. For example, Michael suddenly found himself without company during the day, without the structure of an office, without anyone to have lunch with, gossip with or make coffee for. There was no one to care or notice whether he got up in the morning or what he wore, let alone whether he did any work or not.

Michael also suffered from two other significant losses when he left his job: he lost part of his identity, the part that was a book editor and worked in a smart office in central London, and he also lost the sense of someone else being responsible for his welfare. These losses in particular were disturbing because they echoed similar losses he had felt after his mother's death: then too he had felt very keenly the loss of identity and the loss of someone who had been responsible for him. Being only half aware of these similarities complicated matters further. Not understanding why he was coping so badly with something he had wanted to do – leave a job he wasn't enjoying – made it worse. He felt all the bewilderment and self-doubt that had besieged him after his mother's death, but could not understand why.

If he could have anticipated the similarities, expected the present losses to reactivate memories of the previous losses, Michael might have been spared some of the shock and sense of failure. He could have allowed himself an adjustment phase, in which to grieve for what he was losing by leaving his job, instead of just expecting to be full of energy and enthusiasm for his new life, and being angry and disappointed with himself for not being.

While Michael's loss was one he had a certain degree of control over since he decided to leave his job, often you will not have control of changes and losses in your life: redundancy, for example, can be extremely painful. However it happens, the loss of professional identity is hard to cope with, and when it comes on top of a bereavement this additional loss can be excruciating.

Jim was 21 when his father died after a long and difficult illness. He and Jim had had a complicated relationship and Jim felt guilty after his father's death that he had not been a 'better' son. He also felt bad that he had not been around more in his father's illness and that he was not spending more time now with his widowed mother. A few months after his father died, Jim lost his job in the local theatre where he ran the foyer bar. This second loss in such a short time was too much. He became unable to do anything but sleep and watch television. Very depressed by now, he stopped going out, stopped looking for jobs, stopped talking to his girlfriend or other friends.

For Jim the loss of this job was particularly hard to cope with because it had been an area of strife between his father and him. His father had complained that Jim didn't have a proper job and was not taking work seriously enough. Jim always felt his father regarded him as a failure professionally, but had hoped he would be proud of the job in the local theatre. When his father died, Jim felt a tremendous sense of inadequacy. Irrationally he blamed himself for his father's illness and death, and felt guilty about his behaviour before and after his father's death. His job was his one area of self-pride, in which he hoped eventually to win approval from his father. When he lost the job, it compounded and intensified his already profound sense of failure.

Losing a relationship

Losing a partner can also be the catalyst for reawakened grief after a bereavement.

Mark was apparently unaffected by his mother's death when he was 17. For almost a year, everyone kept saying how well he seemed to have adjusted. Shortly before his mother died he had started going out with Jessica and she had stuck by him, being loving and supportive during the months after his mother's death. People often remarked that Jessica even somewhat resembled Mark's mother. When Jessica finished the relationship after about a year, Mark was completely devastated. All the feelings he had not expressed after his mother died now came out. Jessica had somehow replaced his mother in his mind and heart, and made it possible to avoid grieving for her. When he lost Jessica too, it released a storm of grief.

As with losing a job or a house, it is vital to recognize what you are losing when a relationship ends, and to allow yourself to mourn for it. It is equally vital not to pretend it has no connection with other losses in your life that have gone before.

Happy changes

Sometimes the changes in your life will be happy occasions, such as Christmas or birthdays or weddings. Even so they may still awaken sad memories and painful feelings of loss. A Christmas spent in the absence of one of your parents is bound to be the cause of mixed emotions, however much happiness there also is, simply because the absence will remind you of the death and of previous Christmases when that parent was there. Even happy occasions can involve loss. *Any* event that involves the gain of something new will involve also the loss of something old. Change involves loss, even when it is change that is wanted and joyful, and loss in any circumstances will stir up feelings related to other losses.

Marriage is the obvious and most dramatic example, whether it is the marriage of siblings or parents. Why do brides' mothers traditionally weep at weddings? Not just for joy, that's for sure. They are crying also for the loss of their little girls, for the loss of sexual innocence, for the loss of their own prime position in their daughters' lives, and for the loss of their own youth; for the passing of time and with it the passing of their own lives. Similarly, the birth of a child is often accompanied by self-doubt and depression in the new mother, not purely because of hormonal fluctuations and lack of sleep. It is also because of the loss of identity, perhaps the loss of a youthful figure, perhaps the loss of carefreeness.

Change means loss as well as gain, and loss may hurt.

On the day of my brother's wedding, I cried all morning. I was thrilled for him and thought my future sister-in-law was great. But for me it felt like I was losing my brother, as I had lost my father. For an hour or so it felt like a tragedy!

Will is marrying in the autumn. He can't understand why his mother and sister aren't unequivocally delighted. He is cross and rather hurt that they are less than over-the-moon. His sister explains,

> It's not that we're not pleased and we think she is lovely. But it's a sad time of year anyway, the time of year when our father died. And since he died we've been quite dependent on each other. Now it's like Will won't be needing us any more. It feels a bit like we're losing him too.

In the months leading up to my own marriage I was very aware that there would be moments of sadness in the wedding day for me and my family because my father and stepfather would not be there. I would have liked them to have met my husband, and I would have liked them to have been there sharing the celebrations with us. I knew beforehand that I would miss their presence, and at the risk of casting a dampener on the occasion I decided to ask an old family friend to make the speech traditionally made by the bride's father, and in his speech to mention my father and stepfather, so that through a moment of mentioning them and remembering them they would be there. On the day the friend made the speech and spoke with affection and respect about my father and stepfather. This explicit reference to death and sorrow in the context of so much happiness may have seemed distasteful to some, but to me it felt right. The celebration of life and love that lies at the very heart of a wedding was somehow deepened, not diminished, by the acceptance that loss and grief are also a part of marriage. Above all I was left feeling that two people who had had everything to do with bringing me to that point in time, my wedding day, had been included in the festivities, publicly welcomed in to join the party, so that their faces too had been amongst the many smiling faces that day.

Occasions and events that the outside world regards as joyous, but which for you may be painful and difficult, can be stressful and upsetting. After a parent's death these 'joyous' events are usually ambivalent at best, and at worst, they can be appalling, times when your sense of loss may be reawakened. Try not to deny what you are feeling, but to acknowledge to yourself at least that it is entirely understandable in the circumstances. Sometimes it can be helpful to make this acknowledgement explicit in some way, perhaps by lighting a candle in remembrance of your parent or saying a short prayer or reading a poem. A friend of mine draws herself a 'Feeling Plate' when she finds difficult emotions conflicting with events that objectively should be joyful. She draws a circle on a sheet of blank paper and decorates it with images and words that capture all the things she is feeling. She did this recently when she was moving house and found herself feeling very low about it, even though she'd been looking forward to moving to her new house for months. Drawing a 'Feeling Plate' helped her to identify the sources of her sadness: the ending of a phase of her life, the loss of the home where she'd raised her children, the loss of the house where her parents had last visited her before they died, all the memories associated with that home, happy and sad. Getting it all down on paper, within the one circle, helped her to understand what she'd got 'on her plate' at this moment in her life, and also helped her to bring her different feelings into a coherent whole. Sad and happy feelings often coexist. Recognition of sad feelings need not be depressing, instead it can actually make it easier to see and celebrate the joyful aspects of a celebration. Far more depressing is pretending to be enjoying yourself when you're really not.

Coping with loss of control

All sorts of smaller losses in life can rouse feelings related to a parent's death, and an essential aspect of this is facing the fact that we are not and cannot be in control of all the things that happen to us in our lives. This aspect of mourning a death is particularly difficult for young people, because it comes at a time in your life when you need to feel very much *in* control, to feel you are shaping your life and your future, making the right decisions about what subjects to study, what relationships to have, what jobs to apply for, what college to go to, what house to buy.

It is hard to have confidence in your ability to make these kinds of decisions when you barely know what mood you will be in from one moment to the next, when you are depressed or irritable for no obvious reason. This stage in your life is when you take the control out of your parents' hands and into your own, when you take responsibility for yourself. Usually this process happens gradually, sometimes peacefully, sometimes with a great deal of yelling and fighting on the way. When a parent dies, however, you find you suddenly have a lot more responsibility for yourself than you bargained for, at the same time as suddenly feeling far less in control of yourself and the world than before.

Don't underestimate how hard it is to adjust to a new world full of new people, new routines, new surroundings, new demands and expectations, especially at a time when you have no secure base to spring from. Living away from home for the first time, whether alone or in a shared house, can be hard to handle when you are recently bereaved. Time spent alone can be frightening. It is time for your mind to fill up with unwanted memories and painful images. It can also be hard to cope with other people whose problems seem trivial compared with the death of a parent, and who seem to have all the confidence and complacency about life that you now lack. It can be upsetting not to be in your familiar surroundings with your possessions around you at a time when you crave some kind of stability and familiarity in your life.

When I arrived at university, I wondered how on earth I was going to cope with this brave new world when I was standing on what felt like quicksand. It was all right for other students, I thought, they had firm foundations beneath them. My world, in contrast, was fragile, shaky, unreliable. If the 'aliveness' of my parents could not be relied upon, what on earth could? How could I deal with all these new demands when it took all the energy I had just to believe that my mother and brothers and sisters were still, somewhere, alive and well. Some days the effort of believing that was tiring enough to leave nothing over for metaphysical poets and restoration drama. It certainly did not leave much over for making new friends, which I discovered also requires a firm base of self-confidence and *joie de vivre*. I felt wary of the world around me, and envied the other students their easy confidence and casual trust in the world.

For some people, however, making changes can be a help at a difficult time. For instance, it may be easier for you to have some distance and space between you and your family, particularly if you have had to take on a lot of responsibility for other members of the family and have not had room to feel your own grief and loss. You may also find that through work or college you meet people who have also been through the death of a parent, and who can help you cope with what you are going through. 'The laughter and the love of friends', as Hilaire Belloc put it, can be very comforting, and you may welcome a degree of normality in your life, the opportunity to 'forget' from time to time.

Whatever you decide to do, handle yourself with kid gloves through these changes, take smaller steps rather than bigger ones if possible. Try not to cut yourself off entirely from the old familiar places and people. Allow yourself access to them if it helps you deal with new and unfamiliar things in your life. Tell people around you who need to know what has happened; then at least you need not pretend to be fine when you are not – you have enough to worry about without worrying about how well you're pretending not to be worrying!

Help yourself to carry the weight of these additional losses. Allow yourself to recognize the pain of loss and the sorrow of goodbyes, departures and separations, and try to accept that you may well probably feel these things more keenly than those around you.

In Saul Bellow's novel, *Seize the Day*, a character called Wilhelm who is separated from his wife, out of work, out of money, miserable about his mother's death, and not getting on well with his father, says to himself: 'Everyone was like the faces on a playing card, upside down either way.' This is how it is when someone dies: nothing is right, nothing is how it should be, everything is all twisted and confused and turned upside down. A death changes everything. Nothing is as it was. Everything is strange and unfamiliar, particularly those most familiar things like the chair where your father always sat and which now stands in the corner of the room embarrassing everyone with its emptiness. Like the dress which hangs unworn in the cupboard. Like the faces of your brothers and sisters, pale and slightly distorted with sorrow. No one can quite bear to look anyone else straight in the eye. Things that had no significance before are suddenly full of significance – a hat, a pipe, a football. And things that were once significant are now grey with insignificance – mealtimes, exams, the part-time job going at the newsagent. Nothing is unaltered by death. Accepting that change will happen and that after a parent's death certain changes will be, for you right now, extremely painful is vital. It can make it easier to recognize and cope with the changes themselves, and the difficult feelings they can arouse.

Coping with difficult emotions

Saying to yourself, 'My parent didn't mean to die. I must not be angry', is not going to help you very much. Maybe your parent didn't mean to die, but nevertheless they did die and their death has created problems for you and the rest of your family. Accepting that you do feel angry, that you are not happy about all the upheaval in your life, can be very difficult, but feeling this way is perfectly appropriate. Denied anger can lead to depression, which is far more dangerous in the long run. Anger that never ends is not healthy, of course, but anger roused by the immediate difficulties you are now facing is a normal and helpful response. *Of course* you are angry.

One useful technique for dealing with anger is an exercise called 'How Dare You!' On a piece of paper simply write down everything you can think of that is making you angry. Don't think too hard, just let the words come into your head and write them down. They need not even be thoughts associated explicitly with death. Anything is fine, so long as each sentence you write begins with the words, 'How dare you ... ' 'How dare you die! How dare you leave us! How dare you not make a will! How dare you make us have to move house! How dare you upset us all like this! How dare you upset me! How dare you make it difficult for me to revise for my exams! How dare you ruin my love life! How dare you shake my life upside down like this. ... ' Whatever comes to mind, put it down. Once you've done that, tear your list in half, and in half again, and into the smallest pieces you can, and then throw the pieces away! A variation of this exercise works in exactly the same way except that you start each sentence with the words 'It's just not fair ... '.

These exercises can be very cathartic, a physical and symbolic way of letting go of anger. You will almost certainly find that the anger turns instead into other feelings, such as indignation, sadness, regret or guilt. You will probably also find that the anger you may have feared was so great it would engulf the world is actually not so terrifyingly vast. Bottled up anger seems to get bigger and bigger; it grows to horrifying proportions in the darkness of the heart. If you can just risk letting it out into the open for a bit it will exhaust itself, simmer down and stop.

Don't be frightened of anger. Undoubtedly it is one of the more difficult and distressing emotions bereavement will throw at you, but try to accept it and trust that it is there for good reasons. Try to find non-destructive ways of expressing it. If you can acknowledge your feelings, you can decide what you want to do with them, not let them decide what to do with you.

Chairs, bubbles and boxes

Another technique often used in counselling is called 'The Empty Chair', and you can do this by yourself or with the help of a professional therapist. A chair is positioned on the opposite side of the room and you say to the chair, as if your parent were actually sitting in it, all the things you have been longing to say to them, from 'I really miss you' to 'I'm furious with you! How could you do this to me?' My younger sister developed her own version of 'The Empty Chair' technique. She has a book in which she writes letters to her father whenever she feels the need. Sometimes they are sad letters, sometimes angry letters, sometimes funny ones. It is a valuable way of remaining in communication with her father when there are things she finds she still needs to say to him.

Therapist Peta Hemmings has described how she uses snowstorm toys to help younger children express and work through their feelings of broken trust in the world. 'The glass bubble represents the known boundaries of the world/family. The loss tips everything upside down, and it takes a long time for the elements of that event to subside. ... The slightest knock can send those elements swirling around again.' Having a visual representation of what you are inwardly experiencing or have experienced in the past, particularly if it was before you were able to express yourself easily in words, can be immensely liberating.

Drawing can be another useful way of sorting out your feelings and thoughts. Alan Silberberg found that doodling images helped him to process his feelings long after his mother's death, and to his surprise the doodles turned into the illustrations in his award-winning children's book, *Milo and the Restart Button*. You might like to try a version of this yourself:

- Draw something you worry about
- Draw something you're angry about
- Draw yourself and write words that describe you
- Draw a recent dream you've had
- Draw the ugliest picture you can
- Draw your family as it is now
- Draw your family before your parent died
- Draw something that scares you
- Draw your favourite memory of your dead parent

Clay modeling is another way of expressing feelings in a creative, non-verbal way. Choose colours that reflect different feelings – red for angry, blue for sadness – and make shapes or objects that express happy and sad memories of and feelings about your parent.

One woman I know has a Memory Catcher, a beautiful journal in which she writes down her memories of her mother, who died when she was in her early twenties. She writes things she liked about her mum and things she didn't like; she writes about her mother's hobbies and favourite food. She writes down things she feels good about when she remembers her mother, and things she feels bad or sad about. She also uses her Memory Catcher to write down questions she still has about her mother. Can she still see me? Does a heart attack hurt? And she writes down dreams she has about her mother. The Memory Catcher is the place where she stores anything that reminds her of her mother or helps her to feel connected with her still.

Other people write letters to their dead parent. The letter might include things they wanted to say but didn't or couldn't; things they would have liked to have done or said before their parent died. Sometimes they write to tell their parent how much they loved them and miss them, or to tell them how angry they are that their parent died. They tell their parent what they loved about them, what they'll always remember about them, the ways in which they feel close to them still, what they wish they could still do together and say to one another, advice they'd like to ask for, help they'd like to have. Some people like to keep these letters; others choose to send them heavenwards in a balloon, or bury them in the ground, or scatter them to the four winds or out at sea, or burn them in a special ceremony.

The Ukrainian novelist Vasily Grossman wrote letters to his mother for decades after her death. His mother was murdered by the Nazis in September 1941 in the terrible Berdichev massacre, along with 30,000 other Jewish men, women and children. Grossman was then in his thirties and was working as a war correspondent on the Russian front. For the rest of his life he never stopped thinking about his mother, and he later immortalized her in fictional form in his novel, *Life and Fate*. In the novel the character based on his mother manages to smuggle a last letter to her son out of the ghetto where she is imprisoned and facing the likelihood of death, and amazingly the letter reaches him.

> Several times a day, he would bring the palm of his hand to his chest and pass it over the jacket pocket where he kept the letter. … He knew that he would sooner do away with himself than part with the letter that had so miraculously found him.

As a novelist, Grossman was able to write himself the farewell letter from his mother that he longed for in real life. He also wrote actual letters to her in the years after her death, letters that he could not send, but nevertheless needed to write. On the ninth anniversary of her death, he wrote:

Dearest Mama,

My feelings for you have not diminished one iota; I have not
forgotten you … To me you are as alive as when I was a little
boy and you used to read aloud to me.

In September 1961, on the twentieth anniversary of her death, he wrote
to her again:

Dearest Mama,

It is now twenty years since your death. I love you. I remember you every day of my life, and through all these twenty years,
this grief has been constantly with me …

During those twenty years many people who loved you have
died. You no longer live in Papa's heart, nor in Nadya's, nor in
Auntie Liza's. All are gone. And it seems to me that my love for
you is all the greater, all the more responsible, now that there
are so few living hearts in which you still live. …

Today, as I have done so often during these years, I have
been re-reading the few letters that still remain from among the
many hundreds that I received from you. I have also re-read
your letters to Papa. Reading these letters, I have been crying
once again. … I cry over these letters because you are present in
them. Your kindness is there in them, and your purity, and
your bitter, bitter life, and your nobility, your sense of justice,
your love for me, your concern for others, and your wonderful
mind.

There is nothing I fear, because your love is with me and
because my love is eternally with you.[1]

Grossman's letters are a powerful and poignant testimony to the need of
children of all ages to communicate with their lost parent, to honour the
continuing emotional connection with them long after their physical
death.

If letters are one way to memorialize your parent, memory boxes are
another. In a book or a box, gather memories of your parent using pictures, photos, stories, conversations, ticket stubs, postcards, and objects.
This can be a very moving and positive experience whether you do it on
your own or with other members of your family. It can be a deeply
healing way to talk together, share memories and honour the different
relationship each of you had with the parent who died. Even doing this
with one other sibling can be really positive, or with a friend who's also
lost a parent. A memory box is something you have that you can then go

back to again and again in the future, maybe adding new things when you want.

Worry boxes can also be very helpful. Find an old tissue box. Then on small bits of paper, write out all the things you're worried about. This might be statements, such as: I'm worried about Dad smoking, or I'm worried about Mum going away next week. Or they might be questions that express worries, for example: Did Dad know how much I loved him? Does Mum know I think about her all the time still? Is it wrong to be so sad after all this time? Read the worry out loud and then think of the most reassuring thing you can say to yourself in reply, and if possible think of something positive to do about it. 'I'm right to worry about Dad smoking. I'm going to ask him to stop.' 'It's totally fine to be so sad still about Mum. I can feel as sad as I want.' Once you've got an answer, post the worry into the box. If you can't think of an answer to some of your worries, put them to one side and go back to them later. The more positive and practical ideas you come up with, the easier it gets to think of more. Once the worries are all in, you can say to yourself: 'Here are my worries, safe and sound. I know where they are, so I don't need to worry about them now.'[2]

You may feel a bit self-conscious doing some of these things to start with, but it's nearly always a relief to find there is a safe outlet for your thoughts and feelings. It very much helps to say or write things explicitly, to hear that they are not so unreasonable, that it is not so peculiar to be angry or full of self-pity or frightened. It helps to know the world won't collapse because of the feelings and thoughts inside you. The important thing with all these techniques is to address your parent directly. All the above techniques can be very effective ways of relieving the tension of having thoughts and feelings with nowhere to go, as well as helping you to identify exactly what it is that you are thinking and feeling.

Bereavement does not turn us into saints, and it doesn't turn your dead parent into a saint either. Telling them how much they have hurt you, how difficult they have made things for you, how hard you are finding life without them, helps keep you both human. In the long run it is easier to mourn for a human being than for a saint. It is also easier to *live* with a human being than a saint, and ultimately, when you have mourned your dead, it is vital that you set about finding ways of living with them.

8

OLD GRIEF IN NEW GUISES

There is no present and no future; only the past happening over and over again.

Eugene O'Neill

Accepting just how long the legacy of loss continues to make itself felt is one of the hardest aspects of a bereavement. Long, long after the actual event of a parent's death, the ripples and reverberations are still affecting your life. Sometimes you can feel as if there is no escape from the past, it just keeps coming back to haunt you; sometimes it can return in ways that are hard to recognize and easy to ignore. Often it will seem ludicrous to connect the way you are feeling and behaving with your parent's death, but far below the surface of conscious thought the impact of such a loss *will* still be affecting your life. It will take a long time to learn to live with the death of a parent. Learning to recognize old grief when it appears in new guises can be an immense help.

Like most people, I have experienced the recurrence of old grief in new guises many times since the deaths of my father and stepfather, and, however prepared I think I am, it usually manages to take me by surprise. Seemingly unconnected events have the power to bring all the old pain and anguish flooding back, even years later. Perhaps the most surprising and shocking time this happened to me was when I was 27. My boyfriend (who would later become my husband) had to go abroad unexpectedly on business for a few weeks and we were parted for the first time in our relationship. I was totally unprepared for the agonizing sense of loss that was ushered in by his departure. Left alone in the English countryside, where the spring blossomed into summer, I tipped into heartfelt grief. The sudden departure and abrupt absence of someone I loved very deeply revived all the most painful feelings of loss that I had gone through after my father died *ten years previously*. All the fear of death, of irreversible loss, of my own helplessness in the face of death, and all my fear of the pain of loss reared its head, as terrifying as ever. Until then I had begun to think I had covered over the wounds of my father's death with fresh skin – though still inclined to be a little tender, the wounds were basically healed. How I had underestimated the depth of those wounds! Following my boyfriend's departure I realized that the scar tissue was still new and tender.

Finding myself suddenly bereft of a person I had grown to need and want to be near, I was plunged into despair, felt lost, inadequate, invisible, impotent. I was angry with my partner for going away, for leaving me prey to all these old agonies, for subjecting me to this assault from my past. It was the same anger I felt after my father died, anger at the injustice, the impotence, the fear, the sense of aloneness.

Repeatedly I told myself to be patient, that it was only a few weeks and that he would soon be back, but my mind was not my own; it performed acrobatics I had no control over. When I tried to be calm and rational about my feelings, my mind would somersault and shriek with unkind laughter: 'How can you be so stupid? Why should he come back? Your father didn't. Neither did your stepfather – and he only went for the weekend. Who are you kidding? He's probably dead already.' 'No, no, no, no,' I'd tell myself. 'He's fine, he's coming back.' At which my mind would do a crafty backflip to say, 'There are more ways of losing someone than death, you know. What if, at this very moment, he has realized he doesn't love you anymore?' 'Don't be stupid,' I'd shout back. 'Of course he still loves me. This is ridiculous!' 'But what if … ' said my mind with a little cartwheel.

If my mind was spritely and agile, emotionally and physically I felt as if I had undergone major surgery. Parts of me had been savagely removed and I was less than whole. I had no energy or concentration for anything, roamed listlessly from room to room, searching without even quite realizing what I was searching for. I tried to watch TV, stared gloomily at the flowers outside in the burgeoning summer, could not sleep, could not even eat.

Yet so much of all this was totally familiar. All these feelings and thoughts were there when my father died: the disbelief that makes you wander through the house in a vague hope that you will find the dead one; the numbing tiredness that sends you to bed with limbs like lead and prods you awake with a throbbing headache; the doubts and recriminations that make you think it is your fault that this dreadful thing has happened, that you somehow caused it and deserve it, that maybe if you had been nicer, quieter, prettier, cleverer, whatever, it wouldn't have happened; the fear that you will never be better, never ever be able to smile or laugh again, that happiness for you is a thing of the past; the sensation of being damaged, broken in some way deep inside; the rage, that makes you hate the person for causing you this anguish, for leaving you in this way, for failing to care for you as they should; the surge of emotions, so difficult to face that you either cannot eat with sickness, or eat too much to stifle the feelings that otherwise will stifle you.

My boyfriend's absence, the abrupt dislocation from his physical presence, seemed to me indistinguishable from death. Each time the phone rang I sprang to pick up the receiver thinking, 'It may be him', and sometimes it *was* him. But even then there was pain: the violent collision between the fantasy that he was dead and the proof of his aliveness made me feel I was going a bit crazy; hearing his voice I would be confused into silence, could only think: 'But how can it be him? So he *is* alive?' Quietly working away in the back of my mind through all the hours and minutes of our separation was the certain knowledge that he must have died. I was totally befuddled! My rational brain and my profound irrational fantasies tussled over the evidence. After my father died I would leap to answer the phone when it rang, unable to stop the voice in my head saying 'It might be Dad calling', remembering only afterwards that Dad had been buried a fortnight before. And now there was this other much-loved much-mourned voice on the other end of the line asking how I was, what I'd been doing, and I had no reply other than the unutterable truth: 'Killing you in my imagination and reliving the past.'

Utterly confused by my reaction to my boyfriend's absence, without any way of understanding it other than as a kind of death, I found myself terrified of the possibility that he really might die. I tormented myself with the thought, and felt, once again, entirely alone with these terrible fears. In the same way as I had once felt unable to explain or share or receive adequate sympathy for the father I had lost, I now found myself convinced that no one else could possibly understand how vital *this* man was to me. How could they appreciate how terrified I was that he would not return? And if my worst fears were realized, how could they begin to understand that I had lost what was most precious to me in the whole world? No one possibly could. I was lost once more, alone, terrified.

And there I was, killing him again!

It was as if, ten years on, the death of my father still prevented me from making the imaginative leap from death to temporary separation. In my mind the two were one and the same. There was no difference. Away meant dead, and even though I knew perfectly well that this was not so, equally, with another part of my mind, I knew perfectly well that it was. I was suffering from a severe attack of 'old grief in new guises'.

Much later I came to understand that I was having a flashback to the trauma of my father's sudden death. It's hard to believe that something as common as bereavement can be traumatic in the way that a car crash or a mugging are, but in fact there is plenty of evidence that a sudden and very shocking death can leave people vulnerable to Post Traumatic Stress, and to powerful flashbacks in which they re-experience all the feelings that occurred when the original event took place.

Unlike people who have never experienced a bereavement, I could not pretend that death does not happen. I knew, for a fact – and a fact deeply encoded in my neurological circuitry – that it did: that people you love sometimes do die, that sometimes you speak to a person on the phone at night and in the morning that person is dead. However much I told myself – sternly, fiercely, angrily, even gently – that my boyfriend in all probability would not die, that because it had happened before did *not* mean it would happen again, still it was the most fantastic struggle to silence my overactive brain and still the tide of panic. At some level I was again the 18-year-old, confused, bewildered and betrayed by the sudden disappearance of my father from the physical and emotional stage of my life.

Old wine in new bottles

We human beings are not unlike wine bottles, full of a heady mixture of emotions and thoughts provoked by all the business of the day, the week, the month, from a loving word, a good film, a sad item on the radio or an argument with a friend. After the traumatic event of a parent's death, you can find yourself flooded with feelings, and may well need to put some of the overflow into new bottles. The problem is that these new bottles are easy to mislabel. Instead of 'Bereavement' or 'Grief' or 'Mum's death', you may have stuck on a label saying, 'Wrong job', 'Rotten teacher', 'Drugs', 'Boyfriend' or 'Anorexia'. One of the hardest and most pro-longed tasks of grieving is learning to recognize when a bottle has been wrongly labelled and when you are tasting the same old wine as before.

There are basically two ways in which you may encounter old wine in new and wrongly labelled bottles. First, when events in your life (which perhaps involve some kind of loss) reactivate painful emotions connected with your parent's death and then become hard to handle because they are now emotionally charged far beyond their true significance. Second, when feelings of grief are too painful to be felt in direct relation to your parent, and therefore have to find new ways of coming out. Old grief may come up in new guises in the first months of a bereavement, but equally it may emerge years, even decades, later. Psychologists sometimes call this experience 'regrief', and believe that it is particularly common in people who lose parents in childhood:

Unlike bereavement in adults, which is typically characterized by a discrete mourning period that abates over time, the loss of a parent at an early age informs and becomes incorporated into a bereaved child's personality, identity and world view. The general childhood bereavement literature suggests that grief does not end for children and might more aptly be described as regrief. Thus, it is common for grief to recur in episodic pangs over a lifetime, sometimes as a function of cognitive and emotional maturation, at other times triggered by some emotional or physical cue, or in response to future losses. As children mature, the focus of their grief may shift from missing the deceased parent to lamenting what the parent could have been to the child and coming to terms with the parent's own agency in his or her absence. As well, the manner in which children come to define the memory of the deceased may determine their level of adaptation and coping throughout childhood and adulthood.[1]

As a child, Pippa had craved the attention of her mother, who tended instead to ignore her and spoil her pretty younger sister. When her mother died, Pippa was 16 and her hopes of ever getting that attention from her mother died too. Subconsciously she accepted that from then on she was destined to be the least favoured one in any group. Several years after her mother's death, Pippa found herself working for a difficult, bullying woman who persistently praised her colleagues in the office and omitted to praise her. Pippa found herself re-experiencing all the painful feelings of her childhood, feeling once again the helplessness of the child ignored by her mother. It took a while to make this connection between her mother's neglect and her employer's neglect, and even afterwards it was still very hard to stand up to her employer's unfair and unprofessional behaviour. It was difficult to remember that she was no longer the powerless child, but an adult able to act like an adult, with the power of words and actions on her side.

When there is a large parent-shaped gap in your life, a teacher or tutor or boss can start to fill that space, sometimes in a positive way, as a guide or mentor, but sometimes negatively, as Pippa discovered.

I was lucky in my first job to have an exceptionally nice employer. It was my first experience of living in London and my first experience of living on my own, and I think I did more grieving that year than in the previous three for the simple reason that for the first time there was time and space for myself. The deaths of my father and my stepfather were still raw wounds, but I was frightened by them, frightened that I would never 'get over it', never be 'normal' again. I wanted more than anything to be like all the other young people that I saw on the Underground, in the office, wandering round the shops in Covent Garden at lunchtimes: good-looking, happy, carefree, or so they seemed. Instead I was me pretending. I was me – worried, anxious, insecure, fearful – acting out this idea of how I ought to be. The effort of the pretence was exhausting and, as often happens when people are under stress and working against themselves, I began to be plagued with colds, coughs, bouts of flu, days of feeling tearful and low. I worried about how much time I was taking off work, but what could I do? I always seemed to be going down with some illness or other. One day I met my boss in the corridor and he asked how I was feeling. On an impulse I decided to be honest rather than brave. I admitted that I was pretty miserable and finding it hard to get going again after two bereavements. To my surprise, a look of relief came over his face. 'Oh, I wish you'd told me before,' he said, kindly, 'I didn't know what was going on, I thought maybe you were hating the job or something. I could have been more help to you if I'd known what the matter was.'

Not all bosses are this nice, nor all teachers: often problems at work or school are overlooked or misunderstood through the insensitivity of employers and teachers. But sometimes school or work is a 'new bottle' for the 'old wine' of your grief.

Anna, whose father died when she was in her teens, found the anniversary of his death so difficult to face that she rebottled her feelings of anxiety and distress into dissatisfaction with work. Almost without fail, she would build up to a crisis in her job at around the time of the anniversary, which often resulted in her handing in her notice or getting fired. 'It took me ages to see that there was a pattern to my difficulties at work,' she says, 'and even longer to connect it to my father's death'. Once she had made the connection, however, Anna was able to stop expressing her grief by creating upheaval in her work. This in turn allowed her to find a degree of stability in her life which, with time, made it easier for her to face her unresolved grief directly.

If this scenario sounds familiar to you, stop and ask yourself what the situation at work reminds you of. A bullying, unjust, exacting boss can remind you of a father or mother who also may have bullied you or treated you unfairly. Similarly a critical teacher may remind you of a critical parent. 'She's just like my bloody mother,' you might have said when your parent was still alive, and fought against it. Now, with all the complicated reactions of grief, you might at some level believe that you have to take this criticism, perhaps because it somehow makes you feel close to your dead parent, or perhaps because you feel it is just punishment for negative feelings you had towards your parent when he or she was alive.

Relationships, too, can easily become the new bottle that holds old wine. In *A Secure Base,* John Bowlby describes the case of a man of 27 who became suicidally depressed after splitting up with his girlfriend. He also started to suffer from a range of physical sensations, including a feeling of choking. With the help of a sensitive and alert psychoanalyst, he was able to unearth a long-buried memory of witnessing his mother's attempted suicide when he was a small boy. Certain similarities in the way he broke up with his girlfriend had triggered a memory of this traumatic event.

If losing a lover can stir painful feelings and memories after twenty-five years, it is not so strange to be reminded of the death of a parent only two or three years back when you split up with a partner, especially if there are difficult thoughts and feelings that you have until now avoided.

Not long after Sian's father died, she also split up with her boyfriend. They had been together for almost ten years, since they were teenagers, and although the relationship had its problems, she always thought they would stay together. One day, however, she came home to find her boyfriend had moved out. These two sudden and totally unexpected losses so close to each other were terrible for her. She felt as if her whole life were crumbling around her. She was furious with her boyfriend for leaving her when she needed him, but at the same time she still believed he would come back to her. Sian justified her hopes that her boyfriend would return by reasoning that her father's death had perhaps triggered painful memories for him because his own father had died when he was a child. It was his bereavement that he was running away from, she reasoned, not their relationship. Whatever his reasons for leaving, the boyfriend never did come back and he left Sian with two losses to come to terms with, which she did only with some difficulty. All her negative, hostile feelings she attributed to her boyfriend, while all her positive, sad feelings she directed towards her father. She could believe that her father was dead, but she could not believe that her boyfriend had left her. The truth of the matter was that she needed to believe, and to come to terms with, both these losses.

Sian found, and this is not uncommon, that when there are unresolved and complicated feelings for the person who has died, it is possible to face some of those feelings about that person and the death, but others get stashed away until another target can be found for them. In Sian's case, many of the feelings of rage and hostility and contempt that she felt towards her boyfriend were feelings she had long harboured towards her father, but which she could not admit to feeling.

In Jane Austen's novel *Northanger Abbey*, 17-year-old Catherine learns that the mother of her friend, Eleanor, had died some years before. 'Her death must have been a great affliction!' Catherine says to her friend. '"A great and increasing one," replied the other, in a low voice. "I was only thirteen when it happened; and though I felt my loss perhaps as strongly as one so young could feel it, I did not, I could not then know what a loss it was."' Eleanor's words show an insight most of us unfortunately lack about the continuing effects of a parent's death. Recognizing the influence of the past in the patterns of the present makes it easier to separate past from present. Realizing how new problems in your life may be related to old ones is the first vital step towards making sense of things, the first step towards labelling your wine bottles properly.

Nevertheless it is shocking how an event that takes place years after your parent died can catapult you right back into the fears and anxieties of the time immediately surrounding the death, feelings you thought you'd put behind you for ever. It helps to understand that these may be 'old' feelings, that your reactions may be more appropriate to then than now. The experience may not be any the less intense or harrowing or real for that little bit of calm rationality that can say, 'This is old business'. The force and power and resilience of these irrational frightening thoughts can be terrifying, and the difficulties that exist in overcoming them are very real, even when you know them to be irrational and unrealistic. Even when you can argue with yourself, can understand the source of these thoughts and feelings, they can still hold you in their grip. But it does help to be prepared for the resurrection of these old painful feelings, because if you can anticipate them it allows you to prepare a little for them, to find ways of cushioning the blow of those thoughts and feelings, and to protect yourself from their impact. Most importantly, recognizing and anticipating the real roots of these emotions makes them easier to live with, and in turn makes it easier not to punish yourself for feeling miserable, angry, resentful, confused. You can, at the very least, not add guilt and shame to an already seething pot of feelings.

Repeating patterns

Psychologists and psychoanalysts have long recognized the way in which people repeat patterns in their lives. As the philosopher George Santayana put it: 'Those who cannot remember the past are condemned to repeat it.'

The particular pattern of repetition will be different for everyone: for some people it is the boss they simply cannot please no matter how often they change jobs, or the relationships that all break down after six months; for others it can be a specific habit, like always getting drunk before an important event, or habitually getting caught speeding, or continually falling out with friends. Until we recognize the underlying cause of these patterns of behaviour, we can find ourselves unconsciously recreating situations in which we force ourselves to go through the same emotions.

It is not unlike the way a musician practises a difficult phrase of music: unless the musician stops and sorts out why she or he can't play a particular bit, works out whether it is the fingering, the timing or the articulation that is causing the problem, she or he will continue to stumble and falter at that same point. Stopping and practising once may not be enough to solve the problem immediately; maybe it will be necessary to go over a passage or phrase many times before it can be managed without faltering. Life is like this too.

It took one man fifteen years to work out the 'passage' that he repeatedly stumbled at. It wasn't until his personal life had got into serious disarray that he was forced to stop and look at what was happening. Only then did he begin to understand how the element of pain involved in loving someone had become intolerable after his mother died when he was 17. In a desperate and futile attempt to protect himself from pain, he had shut out the risk of further suffering by ending the relationship he was in at the time of her death. When a few years later his father remarried and he 'lost' him too, he again slammed down the emotional hatches, ending the relationship he was then in. Over the next ten years all his relationships had got stuck at the first sign of difficulty: when the going got tough, when love involved pain, he found it intolerable and refused to go on. It gave him a sense of power at a time when he felt powerless and out of control. It was a pattern he was repeating unconsciously, and until it led to the breakdown of his marriage, it was a pattern that in some senses served him quite well.

Angela 'practised' her fears too, but was able to work out the problem before things got out of hand. She started going out with her boyfriend a year after her father died. He was kind and affectionate and helped her recover her confidence in herself and in life – up to a certain point. That point was his passion for rock climbing. Every other weekend or so he went off, leaving Angela convinced it was the last time she would see him. She lived his death in her imagination every second that he was away. When he came back, safe and sound, she was exhausted with worry and in a state of silent rage that he had inflicted so much pain on her so unnecessarily. She hated herself for not 'coping' and blamed herself for her suffering as much as she blamed him. Eventually she began to see that in the circumstances it was not surprising that she was so frightened by his rock climbing, and that what *was* wrong was putting herself through such an ordeal on a regular basis. In the context of her father's recent death, she could not be expected to cope equably with these separations. Her boyfriend would not or could not understand how distressing his risk-taking was for her, and in the end he and Angela decided to go their separate ways.

Her fear and distress was the old wine of her grief in the new bottle of his rock climbing. Recognizing that her feelings were related to an earlier event made it easier for Angela to understand and accept her fear and find ways of looking after herself instead of needlessly hurting herself further. She too turned her back on a relationship but in her case it was for positive reasons.

The Secret Garden by Frances Hodgson Burnett is about two bereaved children whose lives have 'got stuck'. Colin is an invalid and terrified he is going to die. He is unable to tolerate any difficulties or obstructions and when they do occur is thrown into a hysterical frenzy. He is a child assaulted by the past, his tantrums express the fear-filled panic of a child whose mother has died and whose life has fallen apart. He says, at one point, 'I wish I had died too.' But in the course of the story, he learns that there is a way through these moments of fear, that old painful feelings must be looked at and that obstacles in life are also challenges that can be transforming in positive ways. Through his friendship with Mary, he begins to live with enthusiasm for the present and hope for the future. The locked secret garden, which the children discover and gradually bring to life, is a powerful image for the 'stuck' state that many bereaved people confront in themselves. Unless the symbolic tangle of thorny bushes in the secret garden are pruned, or the problematic sequence of notes in a piece of music looked at and gone over, the legacy of bereavement can continue to trap you for years and years, sometimes in dangerous and life-threatening ways.

It can be tempting – and sometimes necessary – to try to avoid the perplexing symptoms of grief, and people often do: they change job a lot; they change partner a lot; they go abroad; they move house every few months. Any substantial degree of commitment, be it to a place, a job, or a person, rouses the painful possibility of loss. Having something makes you think how it would be not to have it. If in the past you decided that loss was unbearably painful and therefore all future pain should be avoided by never risking loss, to a certain extent you are protecting yourself from difficult emotions, but inevitably you lose out, because by avoiding the consequences of losing anything, you avoid also the con-sequences of ever really having anything. History and psychology books are full of accounts of people whose lives have remained empty of love, fulfilment and happiness because they could not bear the possibility of their opposites: loss, loneliness, sadness. The irony is that they ended up with those feelings anyway without having had the pleasure of their opposites. As Santayana put it, 'Only people who avoid love can avoid grief. The point is to learn from it and remain vulnerable to love.'

Unlike homework or games lessons or office parties, grief cannot be avoided without paying a price. There is no question of avoiding grief. People sometimes imagine they can. They shut down inside, freeze up, simply refuse to let themselves feel the pain of their loss, the anger, sadness, confusion, guilt. They button themselves up and stiffen their upper lip and say, 'Well, can't sit around here moping', or 'Dad would hate me to fail my exams', or 'It's not so bad, other people have far worse things happen to them', or 'No time to think about my problems, I've got to make sure the rest of the family is all right now that Mum is dead.'

All these thoughts may be appropriate at some point, but perhaps not right now. Using thoughts like these to keep difficult emotions under control is a short-term strategy for survival, not a long-term route to recovery. Time tends to reveal that people who have gained control in this way have not succeeded in 'getting over it', but only in delaying the moment when they must grieve. The moment when the stored-up grief wells up and bursts out is more, not less, painful for the intervening years, as William Styron, who wrote the novel and screenplay for the film *Sophie's Choice*, poignantly describes in his book, *Darkness Visible*. When he finally gave up drink, after years of using it as a protection against the inner world of troubling emotions and thoughts, he was catapulted into a nervous breakdown. He was then in his sixties, but in the months following the breakdown, he began to attribute a lifetime of alcohol abuse and recurrent depressions – which although he denied them, had gathered like storm clouds – to his mother's death when he was a teenager. He writes of 'an insufferable burden, of which rage and guilt, and not only dammed-up sorrow, are a part'. These, he says, were 'the potential seeds of self-destruction'. He goes on:

> ... disorder and early sorrow – the death or disappearance of a parent, especially a mother, before or during puberty – appears repeatedly in the literature on depression as a trauma sometimes likely to create nearly irreparable emotional havoc.

It is important to realize that while grief may emerge in new guises in the first months of a bereavement, equally it may come up years, even decades, after a parent's death. It is this old grief that plays such havoc in people's lives when it appears later on in new and strange ways, in the places and at the times we least expect it to.

Hurting yourself to avoid the pain

Trying to avoid the pain of loss is one of the key reasons why old grief so often appears in new guises. People are extraordinarily adept and ingenious in their attempts to shut out painful feelings, but painful feelings are just as adept and ingenious at making themselves felt. Often the person who gets harmed, unwittingly, by this struggle is you.

It is extremely hard to feel loving and kind towards yourself when a parent has died and when the world around you seems to be so cruel and uncaring. Perhaps there is even a kind of comfort to be had from being the one to inflict the pain, rather than having it inflicted: at least you have a sense of control, instead of the dreadful feeling of impotence that so often comes in the wake of a parent's death.

This desire and need to feel in control, and thereby regain at least some sense of power over your life, is always keen after a bereavement, but it is particularly so in your teens and twenties when issues of power and control – of self-efficacy – are all-important.

It is not surprising that when a parent dies, the need for some control of your life becomes even greater, and this makes it all the more terrifying to be so *out* of control, to have thoughts and feelings taking over at the most inconvenient and unexpected times. As one woman put it six months after her mother's death: 'The big pressures in my life aren't the problem. I can cope with those. It's when I'm washing up or just sitting quietly after supper that it really hurts.'

However much you long to be spared these awful moments of surging pain and sorrow, it is very important to accept that trying to shut them out is not going to help matters in the long term, if doing so means suppressing feelings that need to be expressed. The result is often you succeed in 'conquering' grief only by finding other ways of hurting yourself. Recognizing that you may be trying to control the uncontrollable is a big step towards helping yourself after a parent's death. And recognizing the ways in which you may be trying to get that control over painful, unwanted emotions is of course vital.

Hurting yourself with drugs

Judith was 17 when her father died. She spent the next six months drinking heavily and taking drugs. She did not mind feeling out of control as long as she was the one to decide when and how it happened. What she could not tolerate was the involuntary 'out-of-control' caused by her father's death and her reaction to it. It seemed as if she had a drug problem; what she really had was a grief problem.

Jamie, aged 15, used drugs in a different way but for the same ultimate purpose: to feel in charge of a situation that was painfully out of his control. Jamie's father had died several years previously and he had suffered from terrible nightmares for some time afterwards. Although he had brothers and sisters, Jamie was the youngest and his mother's favourite, and after his father's death they became closer still. The problems began when his mother decided to remarry.

About the time that her future husband moved in, Jamie began to get involved with drugs, supplying cannabis to his friends, and enjoying the money, status and power this brought him. His mother, immersed in her new relationship, failed to notice that her son was rather well off for a schoolboy who didn't even have a Saturday job, nor did she remark on how many friends he suddenly seemed to have acquired. Two days before his mother's wedding, Jamie was arrested for dealing and possession.

Later, in court, the probation officer linked his father's death and his mother's remarriage as prime causes, a connection neither Jamie nor his mother had made themselves until then, but which in retrospect began to make sense. Her impending marriage brought up painful feelings of helplessness, abandonment and rejection in Jamie, but he was unable to express his feelings directly, either to himself or anyone else. Instead he turned his attention away from his family to the world of his friends and looked there for the approval and affirmation he craved and seemed about to lose.

Jamie hadn't intended to get so involved with drugs, but they sucked him in, gave him the impression of taking possession of them as they, in reality, took possession of him. At first it seemed the perfect solution to his problems: a way of fending off his diminished importance in his mother's life when for so long he had been all-important to her. Drugs seemed to offer him a way of overcoming the panicky sensation of being insignificant, invisible, pushed out. Instead, they made people want to see him, people treated him as if he mattered, as if he were important. He was suddenly somebody. He was no longer the helpless 15-year-old who had lost his father and was now about to lose his mother, but someone with authority, power, money, status. He was in control. But looked at another way, Jamie was not at all in control. Long before the police caught up with him, he was a prisoner to a similar fear of being helpless and abandoned that Judith experienced. It was a vicious circle which in some ways he had created for himself.

Erle went to live with his grandparents after his father's death when he was a teenager. He describes being 'looked after in a practical way', but internalized feelings of grief and anger remained locked inside and inhabited an inner world that was dark and bleak. At school he remained hardworking and compliant, but inside he felt like a 'rebel without a cause'. In his twenties and thirties he suffered from prolonged bouts of alcohol and drug addiction and subsequent periods of rehab. Only when his life was in total ruin did he finally stop and begin to grieve.[2]

Hurting yourself with sex

Some people try to gain control of their pain not through drugs or alcohol, but through sex. Sex can be a way of feeling close to someone. The feeling of being desired can be intoxicating. The feeling of desiring someone else is similarly revitalizing. The physical proximity of another person's body can be extremely comforting. The sensation of a pair of arms encircling you, the warmth of another person's flesh, the smell of their skin, can shut out the feeling that the world is a cold, hostile place. The physical presence of another person can make you feel more substantial and less fragile in a world that has become unreliable, uncertain, dangerous even.

Physical affection is profoundly necessary. Studies have shown that simply embracing for as little as 20 seconds can boost oxytocin levels in the brain, the so-called 'love hormone' that is also released in mothers when they breastfeed their babies, and in groups of footballers when they warm-up before a match. It's the hormone that makes us feel connected and bonded to other people. Few better ways exist to ease the ache of loneliness. Having someone there who wants you, desires you and compliments you can be very important when you are feeling abandoned, and – as people often do after a bereavement – somehow contaminated and to blame. Physical affection can stop the unpleasant sensation of having some disease that other people are afraid of catching if they get too close: the disease of unhappiness, the disease of death. When people seem to be looking at you with an expression in their eyes that says, 'I'm very sorry for you, but don't come too near', it can be incredibly sustaining to feel physically wanted, to find that people want to get near to you after all.

The physical presence of another person is not only comforting, it is also distracting. Another person's body against yours, another person's hands on your skin, the heady feelings of desire: all these distract you from the muddle in your head, the troubling chaos of emotions. Sex can even counteract the numbness that follows the death of a parent. Physical contact can make you feel alive again, which can be very reassuring.

The problems start when physical affection and sex get confused, and sex becomes the *only* way in which you can feel, the only thing that reawakens sensation, so that you begin to crave it like a drug; it becomes a fix you are dependent on.

After her mother's death, when she was 19, Alison became very promiscuous. She seemed to need sex: it made her feel normal, it made her feel real, it made her feel wanted. Most of all, it made her *feel*. The more men desired her, the more dependent she became on sex. It gave her a sense of power at a time in her life when she felt powerless. It also gave her the sense that her own life had not stopped with her mother's death, but that she, Alison, was continuing to live. She knew that there was a destructive element in her quest for physical sensation: not only did she rarely find lasting physical satisfaction or emotional solace in the men she went to bed with, she also seemed particularly drawn to people she did not know and whom it was actually quite risky to sleep with, frequently they were men with a history of bisexuality or promiscuity. The greater the risk, the greater the attraction. It was as if in her apparent quest for life and feeling, Alison also was seeking a kind of destruction. She was at some level not healing herself but harming herself – and she knew it, but could not stop. In the short periods when she was without a boyfriend, Alison would become beside herself with loneliness, self-hatred and feelings of failure. Before very long she would find someone new on whom to pin all her hopes of survival and rejuvenation, someone who would bring her to life by filling her with desire.

This pattern of behaviour went on for some time, and her love life was a source of amazement and concern to those who cared about her. Alison herself was vaguely aware that there might be some connection between her behaviour and her mother's death, but dismissed the idea because in other respects she had coped well with the death and the subsequent upheavals in her family. It was only after a prolonged bout of depression that Alison decided to have some counselling and at last began to recognize and understand the connection.

Through the counselling sessions she discovered that she was carrying with her not only the positive memories she had of her mother, but also memories of a woman who could be highly critical of her daughter, disapproving and censorious, often not talking to her for days on end. In particular her mother had frowned on Alison's boyfriends, frowned on any suggestion that her little girl was turning into a sexual woman. Her mother's death when she was a teenager and just beginning to explore her sexuality was in a sense a conclusive rejection of the adult self

Alison was becoming. Alison began to see how she had often gone against her mother's wishes with regards to her choice of boyfriend, but that her mother's approval had nevertheless mattered greatly. Now that her mother was dead, who was to give her guidance? She had to carry around inside not only the judging critical voice of her mother, but also her own voice busily rejecting her mother's opinion. Sex for Alison was a way of asserting her independence and punishing her mother for having died. Through sex she could say, 'I can do what I like. I can make up my own mind', and at the same time, 'I can't choose. I am helpless and hopeless without you. I need you.'

Alison also began to understand how her boyfriends had fallen into two quite different categories: on the one hand there were the solid, reliable, steady types, and on the other there were the unpredictable, unreliable, dangerous types. The counsellor asked her, what did she want: a steady, reliable father, or an exciting lover? In Alison's mind, there was no room for the partner who combined these attributes because through her affairs she was playing out two different roles: the girl who deserved to be cared for or the girl who deserved to be punished. Sex can be life-affirming, but it can also be a destructive, aggressive, hostile act. The existence of rape is the extreme proof of the possibility for aggression in sex. Both women and men can use sex as a weapon. Sometimes they use it against the other person, sometimes they use it against themselves.

Alex had a stream of girlfriends after his mother died, never staying much more than one night with any one of them. For him, casual sex served a number of functions: it was a way of trying to get back to some warm safe place where he could for a while forget himself, be relieved of himself, relieved of consciousness; it was also a way of distracting himself: the chase was exhilarating and all-engrossing, but once he'd slept with the current object of his desire, all the excitement was gone and he'd have to start again with someone else. Sex made him feel powerful, it made him feel attractive, wanted, irresistible, important, successful. Filled with his own desire, and his awareness of the girl's desire for him, he could shut out, briefly, all the troubling feelings of helplessness, powerlessness and insignificance that his mother's death roused in him.

Sex also, and quite unconsciously, was a way of punishing his mother for dying. Alex was not easily angered. He had a reputation in his family for being patient and sweet-tempered. Nevertheless his mother's death left him feeling abandoned, bewildered and terribly hurt. He was angry with life for doing this to him, angry with his mother for dying and leaving him, for hurting him, and for hurting his father and sister. By hurting other women, by showing how little he cared about their feelings, how insignificant they were to him, he was trying to show himself that he could be unaffected by his mother's death, that he could in fact hurt her, instead of being hurt.

It was a long time before Alex came to understand the link between his mother's death and his promiscuity. Before that, like Alison, he went through a period of quite serious depression which prompted him to see a therapist. Over the course of several months, therapy helped him to see how he had been using sex to inure himself to the pain and confusion of grief, and at the same time using sex to get back at his mother for having died and left him.

You don't have to be promiscuous to hurt yourself with sex. Tasha started to go out with Martin very soon after her father died, when she was 22. She had not intended or wanted to have a relationship with Martin, but he was very keen on her and because she was grateful to have someone there to comfort her and take her mind off her father's death, she found she had slipped into the relationship despite herself. She was desperate for someone to care for her, hold her, want her, soothe her, but while cuddles were comforting, sex was not. She felt intensely guilty to be having sex at all so soon after her father's death. It felt inappropriate to her. Furthermore, she felt so vulnerable and fragile that the physical act of intercourse was almost unbearable: being physically penetrated made her feel all the more vulnerable. If she felt guilty about having sex, she also felt guilty about not wanting it. She was caught between, on the one hand, wanting to be normal, to have fun and make love like other people of her age, and, on the other hand, needing to grieve for her father. She had quickly become dependent on Martin for his emotional support and was frightened that if she refused to have sex, he might get fed up with her and leave. Another loss, she felt, would be unendurable.

Tasha and Martin stayed together for two years, during which time the problems with their sex life did not improve. Tasha never really got over her initial deep ambivalence about whether or not she wanted to be having a sexual relationship with Martin. She convinced herself that she should want sex, but despite everything her head said, her body would not cooperate. Throughout the time they were together, she had constant recurrences of cystitis and thrush. She also suffered from vaginismus (when the walls of the vagina go into spasm, making penetration difficult and painful). All three of these conditions were related to stress and anxiety, but it was only after she had split up with Martin that she began to see the connection between the timing of the relationship and the constant run of genito-urinary ailments. As she puts it now:

> At the time I was so determined to be the perfect girlfriend, to
> be fun and relaxed and good in bed, that I couldn't accept what

my body was trying so hard to tell me. I made a kind of trade-off: if he hugged me and listened to me and was there for me, I would be there for him sexually. I simply didn't have the strength or courage to say no. I didn't like being boring and frigid. I wanted to be young and carefree. I was annoyed with myself for not being. Now I feel quite ashamed – of how little respect or love I showed myself. If I'm honest, I'm angry with Martin too, for not being more sensitive.

Thinking about the physical act of sex, it isn't hard to see why it seems to offer comfort. It fills you up, literally, or makes you feel contained. Usually, however, a bereavement puts out the sexual lights for a while. You may feel anxious and despondent about the loss of sexual desire, but loss of desire is actually a *natural* response to the very traumatic experience of a parent's death.

Sometimes feelings of grief can be channelled into an increased sex drive, as in Alison and Alex's case, but if you are using sex to mask feelings that need to be dealt with, it can become a very destructive form of behaviour. Try to give yourself time to think about the emotions and fantasies you associate with sex: is it the momentary sensation of power that you like, or the obliteration of worries and cares? Is it the physical touch of someone's skin that you want? Or is sex a way of being aggressive that is somehow 'allowed'? There is nothing wrong with associating any of these feelings with sex, unless doing so is making you miserable and is not satisfying. If so, maybe you can isolate what you want from sex and find it in other ways. Maybe a better way of getting some caring touch is by having a massage. Maybe playing squash is a better way of expressing hostility and aggression.

Hurting yourself with exercise

Even things that are generally regarded as good for you, such as exercise, can in fact be disguises for extremely unhealthy behaviour. Exercise can be a way not of getting fit, but of avoiding painful feelings and keeping up the appearance of being in control of your life. But exercise can become an addiction as unhealthy as any other.

Dale's father died after a long and painful illness when Dale was 20, and in the following years he used exercise to shut out the reality of his loss. He took up running shortly after his father's death, ostensibly for health reasons, but for the next five years became as dependent on his daily run as a heroin addict on his fix. Every morning he had to run for at least two hours; whatever time he had gone to bed the night before, wherever he was in the world, whatever the weather, he ran. It gave him a feeling of calm, of transcendence. Dale also had a demanding job as a junior doctor which involved long hours and hard work. This, combined with his running schedule, left him no free time to reflect on how he felt about his father's death. He was afraid of quiet, contemplative, leisurely time, because it allowed frightening, unwanted thoughts and feelings to emerge. So he ran and worked, and kept a rigid control of those lurking, complicated emotions that threatened to surface if he let up for a moment. But of course he still suffered, not only from extreme fatigue, but also from leaving no room in his life for friends or relationships. Beneath the efficient, highly organized facade, lay great pain and loneliness that he simply could not bear to face.

Hurting yourself with food

Another way of expressing emotions that seem otherwise inexpressible is through food, whether by eating too much or not enough. You are hurting yourself with food if on a regular basis you use food in a way that has nothing to do with physical appetite or nutritional needs, and everything to do with how you are feeling. Anorexia, bulimia and compulsive eating are the technical terms for the various forms of eating disorders, and are methods used primarily, but not exclusively, by young women. This was the method I used to try and gain control at a time when life felt out of my control.

My eating habits had been fairly chaotic since my father's death when I had used food to fill me up and give me comprehensible discomfort instead of the bewildering kind of discomfort caused by sorrow which I had no idea what to do with. I had eaten then to shut out feeling, or at least to provide an easy excuse for feelings I did not like – nausea and anxiety. After my stepfather's death I went the other way and stopped eating, waged war on my appetite, determined to gain control of my own body which was so full of unwanted needs and troubling emotions.

At the same time as refusing to eat, I took responsibility for preparing meals for everyone else. Somewhere in the back of my mind was the idea that if I could only keep people fed, I might somehow keep them alive, make them better; I might be able to fill the emptiness inside them, literally with food, and symbolically with my care and love. But at the same time as I imagined myself responsible for keeping everyone alive, I knew that food was not a magical healing thing, that it could not bring my stepfather back to life, that it could not make people feel better, could not fill the hollowness inside them. After all, it was just food. I was trapped between wanting to look after everyone and make it 'all right', and knowing that I could never achieve this goal, that they had to find ways of looking after themselves, and that all my cooking did not really help them very much at all, however much they thanked me and obediently ate what I produced. At the same time as feeling their lives depended on the meals I made, I also knew how pointless my efforts were, how little difference food made to the vast array of thoughts and feelings caused by a death.

It took me many years to work out that behind my meal-making and desire to care for others was a raging fear of my own emptiness and neediness. I was terrified of the great cavernous gaps inside me and had no idea how to begin to look after myself or care for myself. Instead I turned my attention away from myself and towards everyone else. The person I really wanted to keep alive, and the person I was most scared of failing to keep alive, was myself, but I didn't really know how to deal with that fear, so instead I ignored myself and concentrated – frantically – on meeting everyone else's needs.

After my stepfather's death I somehow convinced myself that if I gave in to my physical need (for food, and all it represented: nurture, care, warmth, solidity, life), I would also be giving in to my emotional needs, which was an utterly terrifying prospect. I would be destroyed, obliterated by my own needs; they would well up inside me like a vast tidal wave and I would be swept away, drowned in their unstoppable flood. I had to keep a tight control of myself at all times, and the easiest way seemed to be through food: I must not give in to any of my needs, starting with the need for food. By determining to be thin and to get thinner, I was attempting two things: first, by giving myself something else to think about, something other than all the pain and sorrow, something of my *own* making, I was taking control of my life; second, by not eating, I was able to tell the world how wretched I was, how frail and vulnerable and fragile. Even if I could hardly bear to see these things in myself, I still wanted to make everyone else see them.

So I got thinner and thinner. And when I went back to university in the autumn for my second year I had lost almost two stones. People were visibly shocked and openly solicitous. And secretly I was pleased. I would not let them forget what had happened to me; I wanted them to feel sorry for me, to see that I was different, special, marked, cursed even, anything but normal, anything but like everyone else. I was determined that they should not expect me to be normal. I would not let them make me hide my feelings away behind a normal, healthy, happy facade. I wanted, I suppose, to punish them with my misery and make them realize how lucky they were. I was envious of their happiness, and jealously guarded my right to unhappiness: I wanted them to feel guilty.

Being thin – and getting thinner – became an obsession and a cause, a crusade almost. It took up nearly all my thinking and energy for three or four years: planning how to eat, how to avoid eating, and how to pretend to eat. I took drugs to suppress my appetite, which left me feeling depressed, so I took other drugs to suppress my depression. Some of these were supplied illegally by friends, others were supplied legally by my doctor. Sometimes I imagined I was winning the battle against grief, at other times it would submerge me. Mostly I wandered about in tears, feeling a complete and utter failure: I had failed to 'get over' my Dad's death, I was plainly failing to shut out my feelings about my stepfather's death, and I had even failed as an anorexic! I was totally useless! Underlying everything was the great unavoidable grief that simply would not be ignored, no matter how hard I tried.

There is a Yiddish proverb which says, 'A man's worst enemy cannot wish him what he thinks up for himself.' The ways that I devised to avoid the much feared pain of grief were more frightening and more painful than the grief itself. Realizing this did not solve things overnight, but it marked a turning point. I still anaesthetized myself with food more often than I'd have liked, and I still panicked when uncomfortable feelings rose up inside me, or when unexpected events happened, but increasingly I stopped setting myself against myself. I gradually stopped setting out to hurt myself, to attack myself. The day I realized that I was no longer using food to justify or avoid feeling miserable, but was instead using it *in response* to feeling miserable was a real turning point.

Learning to tolerate the wait

Alcohol, drugs, sex and food can all be ways of shutting out the world, shutting out awareness of pain and sorrow, shutting out the knowledge of what has happened and the worry that it may happen again. It is very easy and tempting to pretend to be as you think you ought to be, rather than plod along, coping with the painful reality. Drink, drugs and sex are all readily available accomplices in the crime of pretence, but the victim of the crime is usually yourself. While they may make you believe you are OK, having fun, being normal, usually their effect is only temporary, and then you find yourself in the trap of needing more of your fix to get you out of the low left by the last dose.

If you feel that you are adding to your own pain and unhappiness, it can be helpful just to tell yourself that recognizing destructive behaviour is an important start. Try to be patient. Wait for the moment when you have the energy to help yourself, to go out and find what support you need. While you wait, try and accept your feelings and thoughts, without taking refuge in food, drink, drugs or another person's body. Try to 'tolerate the wait', as a friend of mine in her eighties puts it. Learning to tolerate the wait, she says, is the only sure way through periods of intense pain, anguish, loneliness, uncertainty, fear and disruption.

And while you wait, try to protect yourself in non-destructive ways. A drink is not a bad thing in itself, nor is a piece of cake, nor physical affection. Only you can know at what stage things stop being comforting and start to become dangerous. When your own feelings and thoughts seem so frightening and destructive, it is easy to make the mistake of thinking that these feelings and thoughts are what should be avoided, but you can only deny yourself for so long before eventually damaging yourself. However tempting it is to use external factors as a shield to fend off your own unwanted emotions, ultimately, to remain healthy, you will have to put down your shield and take a hard look at what is threatening you. Often you will find there is nothing behind the shield; the thing you have been so frightened of is not behind the shield, but reflected in it. You have to face yourself, and then start to look after that self. Ultimately no one else can do this for you, although they can help a great deal along the way. Try to be as honest with yourself as you can, don't think you are wrong or failing if you feel miserable at times. Try to tolerate the wait and be kind to yourself in the meantime.

9

PATHWAYS TO THE FUTURE

> The future is called 'perhaps', which is the only possible thing to call the future. And the important thing is not to allow that to scare you.
>
> Tennessee Williams

The previous chapters have explained how important it is both to understand the general nature of grief and to take into account the unique circumstances of your particular loss; how doing so makes it easier to accept your feelings and to deal with them; how it then becomes easier to understand and cope when future events in your life cause feelings of grief to recur with renewed force.

Sooner or later, however, the moment comes when you have to approach life as someone who *has been* bereaved rather than someone who *is* bereaved. This in no way invalidates the significance of your loss, or the continuing impact of that loss throughout your life. But it is a vital shift in perspective which marks the fact that life is happening for you once again in the fullest sense. Rushing into this before you are ready can be harmful in the long run, but putting it off indefinitely can be even more so.

Some people find that grief has become a protective layer between them and the world and that over time they have actually grown dependent on the very condition they may hate. Other people find grief 'useful', it lets them off the hook, becomes an easy fallback when they don't feel up to the risks and challenges of life. Sometimes it is hard to know whether or not you have come to terms with your pain and sorrow. Some people force themselves to get on with life before they are ready – sometimes circumstances leave them no choice. This is particularly a problem when you are young: with so many other things demanding your attention and energy, you simply have to leave grieving for later. In that case, it is vital to remember, for reasons explained in the previous chapter, that grieving has to be done at *some* point. There is a critical difference between delaying grief and trying to deny it.

For most people there will come a time when it is right to embrace the future. As Joyce Grenfell put it in *Joyce, by Herself and Her Friends*:

> Weep if you must
> Parting is hell
> But life goes on
> So sing as well

This realization may come to you in a dream, or in a flash of inspiration, it may come out of long and painful struggle. Most likely it will come in a series of different moments spread out across many years. As one man who lost his father as a teenager said:

> For many years following the death of my father, I mourned for something that was missing and I could never exactly identify what it was. Despite never really knowing my father very well, I have come to realize that there was a strong visceral connection between my father and I; in essence, a deep bond of intimacy which transcended the physical and emotional realities of our lived world. But what I can only describe as an inherent part of our relationship was cruelly severed by his untimely death. It is no real wonder then that personal issues relating to intimacy have figured so largely in my adult life. The visceral connection with my father continues to live on between my son and I, a real love that is hard to define.[1]

The fear of fear

In an American comedy act called 'The Two Thousand Year Old Man', Mel Brooks plays a cranky, irrepressible 2,000-year-old man who is being interviewed about his life and times. The interviewer, Carl Reiner, asks him to explain the origin of song.

> 'The origin of song,' says the two thousand year old man, 'is fear.'
> 'Fear?' says the interviewer, very surprised.
> 'Yes, fear. You see a lion coming towards you, you say "help", no one hears you. The lion comes over and bites your leg off.

Now, the *next* time you see a lion coming you YELL, at the top of your voice: "A LI-ON is BI-TING my LEG off. Will SOME-body CALL the COPS." And that is how song began.'

The interviewer presses on: 'And, sir, can you tell us how dancing started? When did man first begin to dance?'

'Well, that was fear too,' the two-thousand year old man replies. 'A man has no eyes in the back of his head to see if a tiger or a lion's coming, so what does he do? He can't stand with his back to a tree all day long. So he asks another guy, preferably a lady, to watch over his shoulder for him. You over mine and me over yours. See! Left a little. Right a little. You got dancing!'

'It seems, sir,' says the interviewer, 'that most things stemmed from fear. Is that right?'

'Yes. Mostly from fear. Yes.'

To stay alive, we must be prepared to feel fearful sometimes, but not to be ruled by fearfulness. After someone dies the temptation to avoid fear at all costs can be very great. But being frightened is not a bad thing in itself; it is not wrong or shameful to be frightened. It is when you begin to fear fear itself, when you become frightened of being frightened, that the problems begin. You may fear dissolution, chaos and collapse, but knowing what you are afraid of creates the possibility of their very opposite: growth, revival, strength. As the 2,000-year-old man explains, fear can have some very positive outcomes.

It may seem hard to believe, but fear is not your enemy but a vital part of yourself, and of life itself. Knowing what is safe and what is dangerous, knowing what to trust and what to fear, saves our lives every day in all sorts of ways. Fear of death and dying, Rousseau maintained over two hundred years ago, 'is the great law of sentient beings, without which the entire human species would soon be destroyed'.

Fear is not wholly negative or wholly positive: if the human being who discovered fire had concluded after the first time that he or she got burnt that fire was to be feared and avoided altogether, the human species would have died of cold and hunger and never made it to the twenty-first century. Fear can make you turn your back on things you need, such as human warmth and connection; it can make you shun the loss of control that is an inevitable part of loving another person; it can make you turn your back on the world, avoid changes and challenges, avoid any situation which might be in any way difficult or dangerous or risky.

I know people who have turned their backs on life through fear. On the outside they seem fine. Maybe they do have nice flats or well-paid jobs or endless streams of girlfriends, but something in them has stopped nevertheless. They create a dangerous kind of control in their lives in order never to feel the fear of being out of control. They won't leave their jobs even though they hate them and don't need the money. They never stay with a partner longer than a few weeks. They can't stand having visitors in their lovely homes. Maybe they drink too much or smoke too much. Maybe they take laxatives at night to control their weight, or live at the pub rather than face an evening alone. I also know people who have simply withdrawn from the world altogether, who do not go out, do not have friends, do not risk anything. Like the hypothetical first human being, who would never risk being burnt, they too are slowly freezing and starving to death.

The most frightening things in life are often the things inside our own hearts and minds. If you dare to look at them and know them and get them out of the darkness into the light you will be all the stronger for it. As St Thomas put it: 'If you bring forth what is inside you, what you bring forth will save you.' It is the fear of fear that stops you looking at, or 'bringing forth', what is inside you; that is the real risk, the real danger, the real thing to be wary of. Fear itself is useful: it tells you about yourself. Not much in life is worse than the things in yourself that you fear, and having once looked at them, nothing else is ever so scary again.

It took me a long, long time to stop fighting (and at the same time denying) my fear, and instead to give it a little room to be. When I found I could do that, I realized that things were not so threatening and dreadful after all. Alongside the fear and despair, I realized, there was also determination and hopefulness. Looking back it makes me very sad to see how hard I was on myself. My whole life in the first few years after my father's and stepfather's deaths was a kind of war against myself, a frantic haze of activity which attacked, and I hoped would subdue, the great army of unwanted emtions inside me. I was like a person besieged, trapped inside myself. And at the same time I was the besieger, the one doing the trapping. I didn't know if I was inside trying to get out, or outside trying to get in. So I just kept building the walls of my battlements and trying to find chinks and holes in the walls – but whether to block up or peer through, I didn't know.

What I did know, was that sooner or later I would have to face all the things I didn't want to face. I would have to accept responsibility for myself and all that involved: accepting that the world was bigger than me and there were things in it I could do nothing about, things that I could only hope to find ways of dealing with, but never ways of causing or preventing. What I slowly, gradually realized was that I was in some ways helpless and powerless, that there were things outside and inside myself that I could not have control over. I just had to let things be, the things I liked and wanted and wished for *and* the things I dreaded and hated and feared. I had to take what there was and work *with* that, not against it.

Taking responsibility for yourself

Trying to avoid painful feelings – or maybe just all feelings – is no way to live: feelings are only avoidable at huge cost to yourself. You *can*, if you wish, choose to avoid feelings, and risk the long-term consequences of that. Or you can try to accept that feelings are not good or bad, though they may be pleasant or painful. Feelings just *are*. If you want to continue in the world leading a fulfilled life, then feelings will *be*. This is not a decision that will illuminate your life overnight; it is a way of being, taking a small step each time you reach a crossroads in your life when you have choice about which path to take.

There are many, many crossroads at which you can exercise choice over your life and yourself. Even when you are convinced you are at a dead end not a crossroads, it is worth remembering a Yiddish proverb: 'No choice is a choice.' But choice is a pain. It involves responsibility, and at the age of 16, 18 or 22, sometimes much older than that, responsibility may be the last thing you need or want. Responsibility is like a mammoth round your neck, never mind an albatross. If choice is a pain, responsibility is even more of a pain. It demands thought and attention. It demands that you look at yourself, your situation, your future, all of which can be fearful things to look at when you are still badly shaken by a parent's death.

One of the hardest lessons of bereavement that I learned was that no one in the world was more responsible for me than I was for myself. People cared for me and loved me and helped me, but no one else was responsible for me. Much as you too might want to eschew that responsibility, in the end it is yours, and you have to own it. Sometimes fully accepting the fact of that responsibility for yourself can come as a relief. It can give you a sense of power, of authority, of having effect. It is a position from which you can look after yourself, value yourself, give yourself what you need. But when it is foisted on you prematurely, it can take a long time to feel and see the good aspects of this responsibility. It is like being made to wear an overcoat – a very thick, heavy overcoat, five sizes too big. It gets in the way. It hangs around your heels and trips you up. It drags over your hands and drops in your food. It is uncomfortable and cumbersome. It slows you down. It makes it impossible to move quickly and easily. Eventually, however, you find it fits a bit better: you can roll back the cuffs if necessary, you can move around in it after all, it keeps you warm, protects you from the cold and damp. Inside your coat you find you are in fact a good deal safer than you were without it. Eventually you even find it is possible to take it off every now and again, hang it up for a while, with no ill effect.

The mantle of self-responsibility is an annoying garment that sits not at all easily at first, but it gets easier to bear. Once you can accept it, responsibility for yourself can bring with it a tremendous sense of relief and of freedom: you are in charge, you are not a powerless child to whom things happen without warning, you are an adult who can respond to the vicissitudes of fortune in ways that will be good for you. You are free to live your life according to your own needs. Few things in life confront us with responsibility for ourselves more directly than becoming a parent, and losing a parent.

The power of memory

If learning to live with fear and accepting responsibility for yourself are two crucial steps towards the future, a third step is recognizing the importance of remembering.

Getting on with your life does not mean you must forget all about the past, but rather that you must make a place for the past in the present and the future. This may sound contradictory, but it is expressed beautifully in a passage from the novel, *Dr Zhivago*. Yuri tells Anna, who is dying, that her death will not be the end of her existence:

> You have always been in others and you will remain in others. And what does it matter to you if later on it is called your memory? This will be you – the real you that enters the future and becomes a part of it.

To take this idea on board involves a radical shift in thinking, because most of us are used to regarding death as an end, a full stop. Even if you believe in some form of life after death, it is still hard to feel that you have any connection with the person who has died. And yet we take it for granted that when someone we care about goes on holiday for a couple of weeks, we will still think and talk about her or him. Why, then, when someone we care about dies, is there an expectation that that person will be somehow erased from our life? Your parent has not vanished, he or she is still with you in your memory, in your attitudes, in your likes and dislikes, in half your genes for heaven's sake! Far from erasing them from your life, the fourth major task of mourning is to form a new kind of relationship with them.

It will not feel so at first, perhaps not for several years, but eventually there can come a point when you will begin to discover that the time you feel so cheated of is there after all. This is a monumental discovery: there *is* time! Not the kind of time you expected or wanted to have, but time nevertheless. You *can* have a relationship with someone who has died. In exactly the same way as a person who goes away continues to be alive in your memory, so a parent who has died does. There is not the same possibility for reunion, but neither is there the absolute halt to your relationship that you might have supposed in the early days after their death.

In the first few years after my father's death, I had the disturbing experience of somehow having him in me, of carrying him in an almost physical sense inside me, so that at times it was as if I were 'being him'. I could catch myself sitting in the same way my father used to, or walking in the same way. It was as if I were doing those things for him now that he could no longer do them for himself. I found this sensation of 'being him' odd and unsettling. His presence inside me was sad and burdensome, as well as wanted. But as the years have passed, this sense of him as a physical presence has worn off. I no longer feel I have to carry him inside me in order to keep him alive, but can find comfort from the memory of him inside me instead. I can still be close to him, still be my father's daughter; it is no longer a burdensome presence inside me, but rather a comfortable space, like a little private meeting place where I can be with him when I want to be.

To find this comfortable – and comforting – room for the past has taken many years. It is thirty years since my father died. I am now the age he was when he died. My daughter is almost the age I was. Life moves on and our understanding of death moves on with it. My father is still part of my life, part of my identity, part of the story of who I am. Occasionally even now I can feel unexpected waves of deep sadness about his death, but they no longer frighten me as they once did. I know from experience that these painful feelings will subside, leaving me with memories and feelings about my father that I am at ease with and welcome.

Before you can live with memories you have to look at them, you have to allow yourself to have them. This is easier to understand in the context of a physical memento of the person, such as a piece of their clothing or a photograph. There was a photograph of my father I was particularly fond of. It showed a side of him I loved: on holiday in a café with a glass of something good to drink in one hand and a spoonful of something good to eat in the other and a huge smile all over his face. This was the fun-loving, good-living, joke-cracking father I had adored. In the months immediately after his death I used to gaze at it and long for him to be alive again. Sometimes I would wonder bitterly if it was the good living that had killed him. But whether the picture roused sad or angry feelings, I was glad to have it there, to be able to see his face.

Later on I went through a stage of wondering if it was wrong to have the photograph of a dead man on my pinboard, perhaps it was morbid. For a while I put it away. Then one day I came across it again, and the lovely expression on my father's face reminded me how infectious his happiness had been and how much I had loved his company at such times. I decided to put it back on my pinboard. I don't *need* it in the way I once did, but I no longer think about taking it down. I no longer feel ashamed of wanting to remember him at times. My father is still part of me and so why pretend otherwise? There are photos of other people who matter to me on the board, so why not him? Sometimes I see the photo and it makes me sad, sometimes it makes me smile, mostly it just gives me a small quiet sense that he is around still somewhere, if nowhere else than in my memory.

You are entitled to your past and to your memories. Unless they are making you ill or destroying you in some way, no one should take them away from you. A sense of the past gives a sense of continuity and a sense of purpose, knowing where you came from affirms your sense of what and where you are now. And knowing where you came from and where you are now in turn enables you to go on into the future. Too much past is a bad thing, but no past at all is possibly worse. To deny what you have been, have had, have done, and have had done to you, is to deny the importance and significance of your experience, of your life, of *you*. A bit of past is a very precious thing and beware of anyone who says otherwise. A bit of past, and the ability to value the past and value memory, not only gives your life meaning, it also gives meaning to the lives of those who have died.

Daniel is in his late fifties, a university lecturer, married with four children. His father died when he was 14. His feelings about his father's death have changed as he has got older, as the years have passed and wedged themselves between him and his original loss. His feelings now are different, he says, but not necessarily easier.

> In a funny way I miss Dad *more* now. I am more aware of not sharing things with him. The events in my life that I would have liked to share with him accumulate over time, and each one reminds you. Having sons of my own completely changed my

view of my father. But the strangest thing of all was reaching the age he'd been when he died: that makes you realize something new about how they must have been in the world. I am now eighteen years *older* than my father. I have passed him in age – and that is really weird. No, his death doesn't get easier with time, it just changes. You never forget, because there are always more things to remind you!

Discovering new things about your relationship with a person who has died, and discovering more about the kind of person they were – and could have been for you had they lived – takes time and is often a painful process, but it does allow your parent to live on through you in a way which is, ultimately, profoundly life-affirming for them and, more importantly, for you. 'There is no death, daughter. People die only when we forget them,' the dying mother says to her daughter in Isabelle Allende's novel *Eva Luna*. 'If you can remember me, I will be with you always.' 'I will remember,' the daughter promises.

At the beginning of this book I emphasized the uniqueness of your relationship with the person who died, something composed of the particular mixture of your two personalities, something that no one else can ever fully understand because it is something only you and your parent experienced. It is important to acknowledge that to yourself in the early days of a bereavement. It is equally important to recognize it later on when you are ready to start living again. Your unique relationship with your parent may be a source of deep pain or a source of joy, maybe it is a mixture of the two; what matters is allowing yourself to remember. Refusing to remember, killing your past, at some level kills you too. To live again, you must also let your dead live, and to do that you must let them stretch and breathe in your memory.

Looking back over the past thirty years, I can see clearly how the deaths of my father and stepfather took the wind out of my sails, how metaphorically 'all at sea' I was for so many years after, without much in the way of rudder, sails or anchor. It is an ongoing source of sadness these two important men in my life have not been able to share important moments with me. My father never knew that I got the place at Cambridge he so wanted for me, that I became a writer not a lawyer. He will never meet my husband, nor my children. There are conversations I wish I could have had with him, about music, and literature, and philosophy, and politics. I would have liked to know what he thought, but never will. Some years ago my oldest brother sent me a photograph of himself, his 5-month-old son, Ben, and our grandfather, Mark, who was then in his eighties. Three generations: 86, 33 and 5 months. The family likeness was very strong, even in the baby. *Already* in the baby! But the photograph made me sad, even as it made me smile, because the absence of one face was so obvious, the missing person so unmissable. There should have been another generation sitting there on the sofa smiling at the camera. Since then I have had two children of my own, whose beautiful faces I search for likenesses, whose emerging personalities I scrutinize for familiar traits. I wish my father and my children could have met each other.

But I find now I can remember my father with pleasure. I can share my memories with him. I can watch how my sense of who he was and who I was then has changed with time. I can enjoy thinking about him. I remember a man who sent me a postcard every morning of my A levels, one of a different famous author each day to arrive before I set off to school: Jane Austen, George Eliot, Keats, Shelley and Thomas Hardy. I remember a man who always sent me wonderful birthday cards – my birthday always fell during term time – and lovely postcards from his holidays in Italy. One of the last was of a fresco of a couple in the bath. On the back of the card he'd written 'Saving water can be fun!' That was typical of a side of my father I loved. It was the same friskiness that often brought on impromptu ditties as we were walking down the street together. Sometimes he might even skip a little! I remember a man who spent infinite care on wrapping paper, ribbons and bows, until the simplest present looked like a work of art; a man who understood that a little girl might appreciate a Christian Dior handkerchief in her Christmas stocking even before she knew who Christian Dior was; a man who adored opera and would sing along to *The Magic Flute* or *Don Giovanni* lustily and tunelessly; a man who enjoyed good food and wine, who on the one hand would buy Tiptree conserve for himself and Robertson's jam for the children, but on the other hand would give me a sip of an exceptional claret so that I might enjoy it too. Going round delicatessens with him was a joy, and nothing compared with his love of a good French patisserie. On camping holidays in Normandy, I just adored the look of guilty delight on his face as he appeared round a corner in some village with a little ribboned box full of *tartes aux fraises* swinging from his hand.

I remember too a man who had a fondness for cashmere socks, and who regularly polished the kitchen floor with them, one toe delicately outstretched like an oversized ballerina; who made the best macaroni cheese in the world, which in my stepmother's absence we would improve still further with lashings of tomato ketchup. Our other culinary game was making Smash instant potato: the challenge was to make it edible by throwing in whatever we could think of, vinegar, paprika, ketchup, eggs, butter, curry powder. We'd usually eaten most of it in the tasting process before the final product reached the table.

I remember a man with a deep appreciation of art, music and literature, which I had little time for at that stage. I remember often seeing him stretched out on the sofa with a whisky and a volume of Keats or Shelley balanced on his chest. I remember so fondly the man who, for my eighteenth birthday, decided it was high time I learned a bit about classical music. Once a fortnight a record would arrive through the post of some major work by Schubert, Mozart, Beethoven or Vivaldi. I see now a man who realized how hard it is to start learning these things, and so got on and started me! The last record – Bach's Double Violin Concerto – arrived ten days before he died.

I remember too with ever-increasing gratitude a man who took me to Rome when I was 16 and brought the whole city, past and present, alive for me. It was the last holiday we went on together. He took me round the ruins of the Old Forum under a baking Roman sun, and somehow made the crumbling walls and half-buried foundations rise out of the dust to all their former magnificence. In the art galleries he showed me how to look at the Giottos and Botticellis. In the cafés he taught me how to sit and watch the world. We got up early to reach the Sistine Chapel before the crowds; we threw coins into the Trevi Fountain, and one night we got lost in the red-light district coming back from a restaurant.

I think I always knew about the sadness in my father, the deep fears and anxieties, but it is through these memories that I have gradually discovered also a man who possessed a tremendous capacity for fun and a tremendous gift for sharing his enjoyment. I have got to know my father better in the years since his death. I feel he is with me still in so many ways.

You too will have your memories of this most special of relationships, both the good sides of it and the bad. Hang on to them. You are the keeper of the past and your memories are the keys to the future.

Into the future

Grieving is hard work, but so is getting on with life. To do so, you have to find the courage to face the three most frightening things of all: mortality, your own self, and the uncertainty of tomorrow. Letting go of grief means overcoming the fear of fear, looking your loss in the face and accepting it, and learning to love your memories not shun them. Getting on with life means accepting that your childhood is over, taking responsibility for yourself, accepting both control of your life and lack of it, and finally – paradoxically – it means allowing the dead to live on in your memory.

Your parent, alive and dead, remains an integral part of your life then, now and in the future, not a chunk of your past to be severed and strewn by the wayside of your sorrow.

I have learnt a great deal about myself in the process of learning to live with a parent's death. I can see, for instance, how I threw myself into wholly unsuitable relationships, and would then be inconsolable when the inevitable break-up came, how I used these hopeless affairs to express the grief and despair I was afraid to feel directly in relation to their real source. I can see how my fear of loss and my fear of my own rage at being 'left' by the deaths of my father and stepfather pushed me not just into men's arms, but into jobs and friendships that had little to do with what I liked, needed or wanted. I did so many things simply to avoid feelings that I was scared of, or because they seemed to be safer causes of distressing feelings than the vast incomprehensible impact of death. I don't exactly regret my mistakes because in a way I had to do the wrong things often enough to *make* myself see that I was doing them wrong, to *convince* myself that I ought to try a different approach. I don't think I wasted those years, but I certainly took plenty of time to reach a stage where I can let the past be, live equably in the present, anticipate enjoyment of the future and feel confident that I have the strength to deal with the inevitable troubles and tragedies the future will hold. I feel able to believe the Jewish proverb that says: 'He that cannot endure the bad, will not live to see the good.' I know that both good and bad, happiness and sorrow lie ahead, and that in all probability they will be endurable.

The death of a parent is not something that fades with time. The person, the sadness of his or her death, the pain of your loss, all are changed by the years, as you are yourself, but they still stay with you. The expression 'time is a great healer' is misleading: time is not so much a great healer as a great transformer. The words used in both the Christian and Jewish funeral liturgy emphasize this: 'earth to earth, ashes to ashes, dust to dust'. Life is changed, life is not taken away. For some the transformation will be relatively quick and smooth, for others it is a long and often painful process. Whatever happens, time cannot erase your loss, but neither will it leave your grief unchanged.

Writing this book required me at times to reach into recesses of myself I would perhaps rather have left untouched. Being aware of the nearness of death to life has made me better able to appreciate and value the preciousness of the moment. Coming to terms with death in general, as well as the specific deaths of people I have loved, has made me if not more willing to take risks, then certainly more aware of the necessity of risk-taking in life, more ready to accept that life is risk, that living is about taking risks, about 'daring to become', or as the theologian Paul Tillich put it, having 'the courage to be'.

Death is out there, waiting for each one of us. However shocking and frightening that realization may be in the first few years after a parent's death, it need not always be oppressive and threatening; instead with time it can release us into the very heart of living. The process of accepting that death is inevitable, that sorrow and pain are equally inevitable, that plans will fall through, that the unexpected will happen, that events and feelings are not always within our control, these realizations can come as a relief. For given those things, what can we do but throw ourselves into the business of life – hopes, joys, uncertainties, upsets, delight, sorrow and all? There is no choice: we must in the end dare to head out into the future.

If nothing else, my encounters with death have taught me this: that we will die and those we love will die. That thorny fact remains, as yet, unsolved by science; it gives meaning to our endeavours and it renders our endeavours meaningless, and in the meantime we must get on with what is both the simplest and the most awesome of tasks: we must dare to live.

USEFUL ORGANIZATIONS

Brake

A charity for anyone bereaved as a result of a road crash, whether the crash happened recently or a long time ago. The confidential helpline is professionally staffed and offers emotional support, information, advocacy, and legal advice. The website provides details of these services and a range of support literature. Brake can liaise with officials on your behalf, and help put you in touch with local specialists in trauma and violent bereavement, or with other people who have experienced being bereaved in a similar way. Brake's free book for children bereaved by road crashes, *Someone Has Died in a Road Crash*, is available through the helpline, and they offer a specialized site to provide advice for carers of children bereaved by any sudden cause.

www.brake.org.uk
PO Box 548
Huddersfield
HD1 2XZ
Helpline: 0845 603 8570 (10 a.m. to 4 p.m. Monday to Friday)
Email: helpline@brake.org.uk

Child Bereavement UK

Offers support and information and a confidential helpline for families and individuals affected when a child is bereaved or when a baby or child dies, as well as training programmes for professionals working with bereaved families. CBC publishes a range of excellent books, DVDs, CD-Roms, workbooks and leaflets. The interactive website includes an online forum for bereaved families, and has a section aimed specifically at 11–25 year olds, with very helpful short films on various aspects of bereavement.

www.childbereavement.org.uk
The Saunderton Estate
Wycombe Road
Saunderton
Buckinghamshire
HP14 4BF
Helpline: +44 (0)1494 568900 (9 a.m. to 5 p.m. weekdays)

Childhood Bereavement Network

Provides useful information for parents, teachers and friends about how to support bereaved children and young people, as well as a directory of local and national support services. The CBN publishes a DVD made by and for teenagers, called *It Will Be OK*, to help bereaved young people understand their experiences after a bereavement. The film is suitable for bereaved children and young people to use in a supported environment. It is also a useful resource for practitioners, parents and carers supporting them.

www.childhoodbereavementnetwork.org.uk
8 Wakley Street
London
EC1V 7QE
Tel: +44 (0)20 7843 6309
Email: cbn@ncb.org.uk

Cruse Bereavement Care

Offers support and information about both the practical and emotional aspects of bereavement. Runs a free telephone helpline and provides free face-to-face support with trained volunteer counsellors. The website contains excellent information for adults, bereaved young people, parents, friends, carers and schools, has very helpful sections on coping with traumatic and violent deaths, and also provides a range of downloadable booklets. Cruse runs a Youth Bereavement Service, and the website has a special section for young people, RD4U, and a DVD, *Ask the Experts*, made by and for young bereaved people.

www.crusebereavementcare.org.uk
1 Victoria Villas
Richmond
Surrey
TW9 2GW

Day by Day Helpline: 0844 477 9400 (9.30 a.m. to 5 p.m. Mon–Fri)
RD4U Helpline: 0808 808 1677 (9.30 a.m. to 5 p.m. Mon–Fri)

A Different Journey

Supports those who have been widowed at a young age through a telephone support network, events and a regular email newsletter.
www.careforthefamily.org.uk
Garth House
Leon Avenue
Cardiff
CF15 7RG
Tel: +44 (0)29 2081 0800
Email: mail@cff.org.uk

DrugFAM

Supports families affected by and bereaved as a result of drugs or alcohol, working with individual family members and carers rather than the user. They offer telephone support, befriending, counselling and local support groups.
www.drugfam.co.uk
8 Castle Street
High Wycombe
Buckinghamshire
HP13 6RF
Tel: 0845 388 3853 or +44 (0)1494 442777 (9 a.m. to 9 p.m.)

Family Lives

A national charity providing help and support with all aspects of family life and family relationships, including those related to a bereavement. The free phoneline is available seven days a week and support is also offered through online chat, textphone and by email.
www.familylives.org.uk
Helpline: 0808 800 2222

Grief Encounter Project

Helps bereaved children and their families get the recognition, understanding and support they need. The website has areas aimed at adults, teenagers and children, and the charity publishes a range of publications and materials, including the Grief Relief Kit, and the Grief Encounter Workbook, an interactive book full of activities to help children and adults learn about and cope with grief.

www.griefencounter.org.uk
PO Box 49701
London
N20 8XJ
Tel: +44 (0)20 8446 7452
Email: contact@griefencounter.org.uk

British Humanist Association

Provides information and assistance with arranging a non-religious funeral. The website has a Frequently Asked Questions page which may help you find further information on common queries.

www.humanism.org.uk
1 Gower Street
London
WC1E 6HD
Tel: +44 (0)20 7079 3580

Inquest

Provides free, confidential help and advice for those facing an inquest. Offers specialized legal advice where the death took place in custody (police, prison, immigration detention and deaths of detained patients), in particular the deaths of women, black people, young people, and people with mental health problems. Advice covers the treatment and care received by the deceased in custody and the experience of bereaved relatives following the death.

www.inquest.org.uk
89–93 Fonthill Road
London
N4 3JH
Tel: +44 (0)20 7263 1111
Fax: +44 (0)20 7561 0799

The Jewish Bereavement Counselling Service

Provides professional, skilled and confidential bereavement counselling to everyone in the Jewish community whatever their values, beliefs, resources and needs who is struggling or having difficulties after the death of a loved one.

www.jbcs.org.uk
Tel: +44 (0)20 8951 3881
Email: enquiries@jbcs.org.uk

National Association of Bereavement Services

A referral agency for bereavement services. Can direct people to their nearest appropriate source of support.

The National Association of Bereavement Services
2nd Floor
4 Pinchin Street
London
E1 6DB
Tel: +44 (0)20 7709 9090

National Stepfamily Association

Offers help and advice to people who find themselves in stepfamilies, and for anyone experiencing difficulties with the new family. It offers a national telephone counselling service for parents.

Chapel House
18 Hatton Place
London
EC1N 8RU
Tel: +44 (0)207 2092460
Helpline: 0808 800 2222

Paul's Fund and Paul's Place

Offers a place for young adults who have been bereaved in the past 2 years, or who are facing a life-threatening diagnosis or terminal illness, or who have a long-term caring role for a family member. Provides grants to 18- to 30-year-olds to cover accommodation costs of holiday break at Paul's Place, a B&B with self-catering facility.

www.pauls-fund.co.uk
Tel: +44 (0)1271 891076
Email: paulsfund11@virginmedia.co.uk

RoadPeace

Runs a helpline for those bereaved by road crashes staffed by trained volunteers who have themselves been bereaved or injured in a crash.

Offers emotional support, practical guidance and information on legal procedures. Help is also available by email and the website provides a road death investigation guide. The charity runs a befriending scheme, which can put you in contact with local people similarly bereaved.

www.roadpeace.org
PO Box 2579
London
NW10 3PW
Tel: +44 (0)208 9641021, administration: +44 (0)208 8385102
Fax: +44 (0)2088385103
Helpline: 0845 4500 355
Email: helpline@roadpeace.org

Samaritans

Provides confidential non-judgmental emotional support 24 hours a day to people who are experiencing feelings of distress or despair, including those which could lead to suicide.

www.samaritans.org
Tel: 08457 90 90 90

SAMM – Support after Murder and Manslaughter

Supports all those who have been bereaved as a result of murder or manslaughter, through a telephone helpline, online forum, home visits by trained volunteers, local support groups, and other activites.

www.samm.org.uk
L&DRC Tally Ho!
Pershore Road
Edgbaston
Birmingham
B5 7RN
Helpline: 0845 872 3440
Email: info@samm.org.uk

Sand Rose Project

Provides free one to two week breaks in a tranquil haven in Cornwall where bereaved families can start to rebuild their lives. The project does not provide therapy or counselling, but works in collaboration with local and national bereavement organizations in England and Wales and is available to families from across the country. Anyone recently bereaved is eligible, although there is a particular emphasis on young families.

www.sandrose.org.uk
PO Box 70
Hayle
TR27 5WY
Tel: 0845 6076357
Email: info@sandrose.org.uk

Seasons for Growth

Seasons for Growth is a loss and grief peer-group support and education programme for young people aged 6–18 years and adults in Australia, New Zealand, Ireland and the United Kingdom. The children and young people's programmes deal with change, loss and grief associated with death, family breakdown, or other forms of separation. Programmes are run over 8 weeks in small groups of between five and seven participants with a trained facilitator. The adult group programmes covers a broader range of life changes related to loss and grief, including unemployment, dislocation, dealing with disabilities, death, divorce, family breakdown and the effects of natural catastrophes. Three different programmes are offered depending on individual concerns. For more details and information about regional programmes, contact the head office or the website.

www.seasonsforgrowth.co.uk
47 Cumberland Street
London
SW1V 4LY
Tel: +44 (0)20 7828 0778
Email: info@seasonsforgrowth.co.uk

Survivors of Bereavement by Suicide

Aims to meet the needs and break the isolation of those bereaved by the suicide of a close relative or friend. Offers a confidential telephone helpline, support information, help by email, group meetings (in a number of locations), one-day conferences, residential events, and information relating to practical issues and problems.

www.uk-sobs.org.uk
The Flamsteed Centre
Albert Street
Ilkeston

Derbyshire
DE7 5GU
Email: sobs.support@hotmail.com
Helpline: 0844 561 6855

WAY (Widowed and Young) FOUNDATION

Provides support, advice and friendship to those who have been bereaved of a partner under the age of 50.
www.wayfoundation.org.uk
Suite 35
St Loyes House,
20 St Loyes Street
Bedford
MK40 1ZL
Tel: 0300 012 4929
Email: info@wayfoundation.org.uk

Winston's Wish

Supports bereaved children up to age 18 who have experienced the death of a parent or sibling. It provides practical help and guidance to bereaved children and their families and also to professionals working with bereaved children through residential weekends, specialized group work and individual therapy. Runs a helpline for people caring for bereaved children and has an excellent website which includes an adult-free zone for young people with information, message boards, downloadable DVDs and podcasts. Publishes a wide range of books and resources on various aspects and types of bereavement.
www.winstonswish.org.uk
4th Floor, St James's House
St James Square
Cheltenham
GL50 3PR
Helpline: 08452 03 04 05. Mon–Fri 9 a.m. to 5 p.m.
General enquiries: +44 (0)1242 515157
Email: info@winstonswish.org.uk

YoungMinds

A UK charity committed to improving the emotional wellbeing and mental health of children and young people. Works directly with children on a wide range of issues, and also supports and provides information for parents and carers. Offers free confidential online and telephone support, including information and advice, to any adult worried about the emotional problems, behaviour or mental health of a child or young person up to the age of 25. Support is available from trained staff through a freephone or by online chat.

www.youngminds.org.uk
Suite 11, Baden Place
Crosby Row
London
SE1 1YW
Helpline: 0808 802 5544 (Monday to Friday 9.30 a.m. to 4 p.m.)
Online chat: parents@youngminds.org.uk Monday to Friday 11 a.m. to 1 p.m.

Additional support

In addition to the above organizations, local branches of Citizens' Advice Bureau can supply details of bereavement services and counsellors in your area. Your GP can also make referrals to NHS or private counsellors and therapists. Many schools, universities and colleges now also have professional counselling services. The following organizations can also be of help in finding specialized help in your area:

British Association for Counselling and Psychotherapy

www.bacp.co.uk
BACP House
15 St John's Business Park
Lutterworth
Leicestershire
LE17 4HB
Tel: +44 (0)1455 883300
Text: +44 (0)1455 550243
Email: bacp@bacp.co.uk

British Association of Psychotherapists

www.bap-psychotherapy.org
37 Mapesbury Road
London

NW2 4HJ
Tel: +44 (0)20 8452 9823
Fax: +44 (0)20 8452 0310

The Centre for Transpersonal Psychology

www.transpersonalcentre.co.uk
17 West View Road
St Albans
Herts
AL3 5JX
Tel: +44 (0)1727 751420
Email: enquiries@transpersonalcentre.co.uk

London Clinic of Psychoanalysis

www.psychoanalysis.org.uk
Byron House
112A Shirland Road
London
W9 2EQ
Tel: +44 (0)20 7563 5002
Fax: +44 (0)20 7563 5003
Email: clinic@iopa.org.uk

The Society of Analytical Psychology

www.thesap.org.uk
1 Daleham Gardens,
London
NW3 5BY
Tel: +44 (0)20 7435 7696
Fax: +44 (0)20 7431 1495

The Westminster Pastoral Foundation

www.wpf.org.uk
23 Magdalen Street
London
SE1 2EN
Tel: +44 (0)20 7378 2000

Women's Therapy Centre

www.womenstherapycentre.co.uk
10 Manor Gardens
London
N7 6JS
Tel: +44 (0)20 7263 7860

Human Givens Institute

www.hgi.org.uk
Chalvington
East Sussex
BN27 3TD
Tel: +44 (0)1323 811662
Fax: +44 (0)1323 811486
Email: hgi@humangivens.com

NOTES

Introduction

1 Rodie Akerman and June Statham, Department for Education Survey, 2010, *Childhood Bereavement Rapid Literature Review.*
2 Dr. Elizabeth Weller, Dir. Ohio State University Hospitals, 1991.
3 U.S. Social Security Administration, 1999, as reported in the *Chicago Tribune Magazine,* 7-18-99.
4 Silverman, Phyllis R. and Nickman, Steven (1996) Children's construction of their dead parent, pp. 73–86, (eds) Klass, D., Silverman, P.R., Nickman, S., *Continuing Bonds: New understanding of grief.* Washington, DC: Taylor & Francis.

1 My story

1 Cheifetz, P.N., Stavrakakis, G. and Lester, E.P. (1989) 'Studies of the affective state in bereaved children', *Canadian Journal of Psychiatry,* 34(7) 688–92. Chiefetz and colleagues studied 16 bereaved children aged 4–17 years old (12 boys and 4 girls) who had lost a parent in the previous 2 years, and found that 69 per cent had symptoms of dysthymia, i.e. depressed mood or loss of interest or pleasure in almost all activities for a period of 1 year. The Childhood Bereavement Study (Worden, 1996) found that 33 per cent of children were at some degree of risk for high levels of emotional and behavioural problems during the 2 years after the death of a parent.
2 Worden, J. William (1996) *Children and Grief: When a Parent Dies* (New York: Guildford Press). The Child Bereavement Study found that children who felt they were allowed to remember their dead parent were less vulnerable to long-term distress: 'Highly connected children were better able to show their emotional pain, to talk with others about the death, and to accept support from families and friends. They were also more likely to visit the gravesite and to observe anniversaries of the death.' They came from families that were rated more cohesive and closer, experienced lower levels of stress, and were more able as a family to talk, remember and relocate the dead parent into a new role within the family.

NOTES

2 First days, last rites

1 Dowdney's review of research on childhood bereavement (Dowdney, 2000) found that specific anxieties are common after death of a parent. These include fears about the surviving parent's safety or other family members; anxiety about separation from remaining attachment figure; somatising symptoms such as headaches, stomach aches, bedwetting. Other symptoms of extreme distress include temper tantrums, hyperactivity, withdrawal. Anxiety is particularly common in very young children, especially when the mother has died, but also common in teenage girls. Reported rates of depression increase with child's age: roughly equal between girls and boys in middle childhood, but more common in girls by adolescence.

2 Worden (1996), op. cit.: '5–7 year olds are particularly vulnerable as cognitive development enables them to understand something of the permanency of death, but they still lack the ego and social skills to deal with the intensity of feelings of loss.' Van Eerdewegh et al. (1982, 1985) studied grief reactions in 105 children aged 2–17 from 50 parentally bereaved families, and found that 13 months after the death, 77 per cent of bereaved children showed high levels of dysphoria (combination of sadness, crying or irritability) compared to 34 per cent of controls. Bereaved children were almost three times as likely to be withdrawn (31 per cent v. 13 per cent) and to have decreased appetite (15 per cent v. 5 per cent), and were more than twice as likely to be having trouble sleeping (19 per cent v. 6 per cent). Overall, they were three times more likely to be classed as mildly depressed (14 per cent v. 4 per cent). These researchers did not interview the children, only the parents. When children themselves are interviewed, studies tend to show up more evidence of distress because bereaved children report more psychiatric symptoms than their parents do of them (Gersten, Beals and Kallgren, 1991). Kranzler et al. (1990) studied 26 children aged 3–6, bereaved in the previous 6 months, and found 40 per cent had serious problems compared to 10 per cent of controls.

3 Worden (1996), op. cit. The Childhood Bereavement Study found that attending the funeral is very helpful and seems to reduce risk of emotional/behavioural problems later: 'Participating in the funeral did not lead to later emotional/behaviour difficulties [while] little or no preparation for the funeral was one of the strong predictors that a child would be at risk 2 years later. Children who weren't prepared for the funeral were more likely to show disturbed behaviour, low self-esteem and low self-efficacy 2 years after the death of a parent.'

4 Raveis, V.H., Siegel, K. and Karus, D. (1999) 'Children's Psychological Distress Following the Death of a Parent', *Journal of Youth and Adolescence* 28: 2.

5 Gorell Barnes, J., Thompson, P., Davies, G. and Burchardt, N. (1997) *Growing Up in Stepfamilies*, Oxford: Oxford University Press.

6 Wood, K., Chase, E. and Aggleton, P. (2006) 'Telling the truth is the best thing: teenage orphans experiences of parental AIDS-related illness and bereavement in Zimbabwe', *Social Science and Medicine* 63(7): 1923–33.

7 Ibid.

8 Worden (1996), op. cit.

9 Silverman, P.R. and Worden, J.W. (1993) 'Children's reactions to the death of a parent', in W. Stroebe, M. Stroebe and R.O. Hansson, *Handbook of Bereavement: Theory, Research and Intervention*, Cambridge: Cambridge University Press.

10 Adapted from Schoen, A.A., Burgoyne, M. and Schoen, F.S. (2004) 'Are the developmental needs of children in America adequately addressed during the grief process?', *Journal of Instructional Psychology* 31(2): 143–8.
11 Irish, D. P., Lundquist, K. F. and Nelsen, V. J. (1993) *Ethnic Variations in Dying, Death, and Grief: Diversity in Universality*, Philadelphia: Taylor & Francis.
12 Rosenblatt, Paul C. (1993) 'Cross-Cultural Variation in the Experience, Expression and Understanding of Grief', in D.P. Irish, K.F. Lundquist and V.J. Nelsen, *Ethnic Variations in Dying, Death, and Grief: Diversity in Universality*, Philadelphia: Taylor & Francis.
13 Worden (1996), op. cit.
14 Silberberg, Alan (2011) *Milo and the Restart Button*, London: Simon and Schuster.
15 Worden (1996), op. cit.

3 Different deaths, different griefs

1 Stokes, J.A. and Crossley, D. (2007) *As Big as It Gets: Supporting a Child When a Parent is Seriously Ill*, Winston's Wish.
2 Silberberg (2011), op. cit.
3 Siegel *et al.* (1992) found that children (7–17 years) whose parents were in the terminal stages of illness showed significantly greater symptoms of depression and anxiety in comparison to controls. At follow-up, between 7 to 12 months after parental death, differences between the groups had become non-significant (Siegel, Karus and Raveis, 1996). Saldinger *et al.* (2003) also found that children who witness physical distress in their dying parents have greater mental health difficulties than children who do not observe such distress.
4 Cohen *et al.* (2002) 'Childhood traumatic grief: concepts and controversies', *Trauma, Violence, and Abuse* 3(4): 307–27. Cohen, J.A., Mannarino, A.P. and Staron, V.R. (2006) 'A pilot study of modified cognitive-behavioural therapy for childhood traumatic grief', *Journal of the American Academy of Child and Adolescent Psychiatry* 45: 1465–73. Brown, E. and Goodman, R. F. (2005) 'Childhood traumatic grief following September 11 2001: construct development and validation', *Journal of Clinical Child and Adolescent Psychology* 34: 248–59.
5 'The Day That Transformed the World', *Independent on Sunday*, 4.9.11.
6 Ibid.
7 Ibid.
8 Personal communication. The Childhood Bereavement Study (Worden, 1996), op. cit., also found that, even in non-complicated bereavements, being able to communicate one's feelings to a trusted adult and having opportunities to talk about the person who died and about the details of their death were key protective factors for bereaved children. Lin *et al.* (2004) found that children's resilience following a caregiver's death was positively predicted by the surviving caregiver's provision of warmth and discipline, and negatively predicted by caregiver mental health problems.
9 Mitchell *et al.* (2006) found that concealing the nature of the death from the child creates an atmosphere of secrecy in the family and teaches the child not to trust his or her own perceptions, memories and observations. Distorted/avoidant communication with the child was a risk factor for subsequent problems, and could result in magical or fantastical accounts to fill the gap, which were traumatic and confusing in their own right.

10 Hung, C. Natalie, and Rabin, Laura, A. (2009) 'Comprehending childhood bereavement by parental suicide: a critical review of research on outcomes, grief process, and interventions', *Death Studies* 33: 781–814.

11 Braiden *et al.* (2009) 'Piloting a therapeutic residential for children, young people and families bereaved through suicide in Northern Ireland', *Child Care in Practice* 15(2): 81–93.

12 Pfeffer *et al.* (1997) studied 16 families with children aged 5–14 years with parent or sibling death by suicide 1–3 years previously. Surviving parent and children were interviewed. 63 per cent of families had children with significant problems of clinical severity; 37 per cent had children showing moderate to severe symptoms of PTSD; 25 per cent of families had at least 1 child with both clinically significant levels of depression and moderate to severe symptoms of PTSD. Yule and Canterbury (1994) found that children who have experienced highly stressful events, especially when death occurs, are at marked risk of PTSD. Tsuchiya *et al.* (2005) found that maternal death through suicide during first decade of life was associated with a 7-fold increase in risk for bipolar disorder in adulthood, but not for maternal death from other causes. For vulnerability of suicidally bereaved children, see also Cerel *et al.* (1999, 2000), Dowdney *et al.* (1999), Mitchell *et al.* (2007).

13 Braiden *et al.* (2009). Cohen *et al.* (2006) developed a CBT treatment for children with traumatic grief where the Post Traumatic Stress responses were impeding their ability to resolve their grief. Children had lost a parent through car accident, homicide, suicide or drug overdose. The program included 12 individual sessions with the child and with the surviving parent, and addressed the trauma and the grief separately. Treatment was highly effective for childhood traumatic grief, PTSD, depression and anxiety.

14 Attempts to evaluate the effectiveness of 'talking cures' and intervention programmes for children coping with violent bereavements have produced mixed results. An evaluation of the Bereavement Group Intervention for suicidally bereaved children by Pfeffer *et al.* (2002) found 'reductions in anxiety and depressive symptoms were significantly greater among children who received the intervention than those who did not.' Sandler *et al.* (2003) found that girls in the Family Bereavement Program showed and reported improvements in externalising and internalising problems after program participation. Brown *et al.* (2007) found inconclusive evidence of the efficacy of intervention, but acknowledge the difficulty of comparing programmes with widely different methodological approaches, samples and attrition rates.

15 Grad, O. and Zavasnik, A. (1996) 'Similarities and differences in the process of bereavement after suicide and after traffic fatalities in Slovenia', *Omega* 33: 243–251. Also, Reed, M.D. (1998) 'Predicting grief symptomatology among the suddenly bereaved', *Suicide and Life-Threatening Behaviour* 21: 385–401.

16 Stroebe and Stroebe (2008) report that both widows and widowers have a higher than average death rate following their spouse's death. Men who lose wives have an increased risk of dying themselves during the first six months after the death, especially younger men, and especially due to accidents. Remarriage buffers widowed men from death. Widows also had a higher than average death rate, but less high than men, and more likely two years after the death. Other studies have found that heart disease accounts for the greatest increase in mortality amongst widowers during the six months post-bereavement; accidents, suicide and liver disease are also common causes of death

post-bereavement, especially for widowed men; and that not only spouses, but parents and sons have raised risk of death from suicide following death of a loved one. See also: Parkes *et al.* (1969); Jones, Goldblatt and Leon (1984); Kaprio *et al.* (1987).

17 Worden (1996), op. cit. Where there was a lot of stress after the death, 13 per cent of children had somatic symptoms in clinical range during early months of bereavement. Higher levels of somatic symptoms were found in children whose families were experiencing a large number of disruptions and changes. These children were more anxious about their own safety and more likely to be having problems with peer relationships. 17 per cent of children continued to have frequent headaches in the second year, girls in particular. 4 per cent of children experienced serious illness in the first 4 months. This was more likely after the death of a father, and when there were high rates of change and conflict within the family. By end of the first year the rate of children with serious illness had *increased* significantly to 10 per cent, but fell to more or less normal levels, compared with non-bereaved children, during the second year.

18 Ibid. The Childhood Bereavement Study found a significant increase in rates of accidents during the first year after parental bereavement, rising from 25 per cent to 34 per cent. Nearly half of the teenage boys (45 per cent) in the study reported having accidents during the first year after parent's death, 1 in 3 of them requiring medical attention. More accidents occurred in households where there was more conflict, and in children who were strongly identified with the dead parent.

19 Ibid.

20 Gorrel Barnes *et al.* (1997), op.cit.

4 Mourning time: the first year

1 Sweeting, H., West, P. and Richards, M. (1998) 'Teenage family life, lifestyles and life chances: associations with family structure, conflict with parents and joint family activity', *International Journal of Law, Policy and the Family* 12(1): 15–46.

2 Several studies show that parents consistently under-report their children's distress. Weller *et al.* (1991) studied 38 prepubertal children from 26 families, interviewing both parents and children 3–12 weeks after the parent's death, and found that 26 per cent of children reported symptoms that matched a major depressive disorder, compared to only 8 per cent according to parental interview. Of these children, 37 per cent were found to be severely depressed, 60 per cent were dysphoric, 61 per cent reported suicidal ideation.

3 Rosenman, S. and Rodgers, B. (2004) 'Childhood adversity in an Australian population', *Social Psychiatry and Psychiatric Epidemiology* 39: 695–702; Rosenman, S. and Rodgers, B. (2006) 'Childhood adversity and adult personality', *Australian and New Zealand Journal of Psychiatry* 40: 482–90.

4 Worden (1996), op. cit.: 'Anxiety levels were higher for girls than boys, and rose significantly for all children during the first year of loss.' The Childhood Bereavement Study also found that social problems and changes in self-perception and self-esteem were more evident 2 years after death. Bereaved children 2 years after a parent's death had more social problems than non-bereaved children, according to both to their parents and their own account, particularly where the mother had died, although pre-teen boys who'd lost a father

also had more difficulties adjusting than other children. Two years after the death, bereaved teens were more withdrawn than non-bereaved teenagers, had more anxiety and depression, more social problems and were more worried about their families. Overall, the Childhood Bereavement Study found that 1 year after death, 19 per cent of Child Bereavement Study children fell into the at risk group compared to 10 per cent of the control, while 2 years after death 21 per cent of Child Bereavement Study children fell into the at risk group compared to 6 per cent of the control. Worden highlights this large and significant difference as one of the most important findings from the study: 'It suggests that there is a "late effect" of bereavement for a significant minority of these school-age children and emphasizes the importance of regular follow-up assessments of children over a longer period of time.'

5 Ibid. The Childhood Bereavement Study found that fathers in general did not make it easy for the child to express thoughts and feelings about his or her dead mother. At 1 year, 78 per cent of children in the study felt they had enough opportunities to talk about their dead parent, i.e. daily or several times a week, were still attached to their dead parent, and able to share dreams and memories of dead parent with another family member. Conversations about the dead parent, however, were much more likely to take place in mother-led families. Children in father-led families had most difficulty talking about their dead parent and had more emotional/behavioural problems, regardless of age and gender. Two years after the death 23 per cent of children still had difficulty talking about their dead parent.

6 Abdelnoor, Adam, and Hollins, Sheila (2004) 'The effects of childhood bereavement on secondary school performance', *Educational Psychology in Practice* 20(1): 43–54. Abdelnoor and Hollins looked at GCSE results for 73 children in UK schools who'd lost a parent and 24 who'd lost a sibling. The bereaved students underachieved significantly depending upon age, gender and parents' employment history, scoring on average half a grade below their controls. The researchers also found a significant rise in anxiety among the parentally bereaved group, who scored 3 or 4 points more on anxiety scales than controls. Children bereaved before the age of 5 and at 12 years of age seemed especially vulnerable to underachievement compared with those bereaved at other ages. Girls were more affected than boys both in terms of school grades and anxiety. Girls whose mothers had died were most at risk in this respect, followed by boys who had lost fathers.

7 Kirwin, K.M. and Hamrin, V. (2005) 'Decreasing the risk of complicated bereavement and future psychiatric disorders in children', *Journal of Child and Adolescent Psychiatric Nursing* 18(2): 62–78.

8 Worden (1996), op.cit.

9 Williams, Caspar (2009*)* 'Adolescent boys and bereavement: a reflexive and phenomenological-narrative analysis of adult men who lost their fathers in adolescence*',* MA dissertation, Regent's College London, July 2009.

10 Normand, L. C., Silverman, P.R. and Nickman, S.L. (1996) 'Bereaved children's changing relationships with the deceased', in D. Klass, P.R. Silverman and S.L. Nickman (eds) *Continuing Bonds: New Understandings of Grief*, Washington, DC: Taylor & Francis. See also Silverman, P.R. (2000) *Never Too Young to Know*, Oxford: Oxford University Press.

11 Ibid.

12 Zisook, S., Devaul, R.A. and Click, M.A. Jr (1982) 'Measuring symptoms of grief and bereavement', *American Journal of Psychiatry* 139(12) 1590–93, cited in W. Middleton, B. Raphael, N. Martinek and V. Misso (1993) 'Pathological Grief Reactions' in W. Stroebe, M. Stroebe, and R.O. Hansson, *Handbook of Bereavement: Theory, Research and Intervention*, Cambridge: Cambridge University Press.

13 Worden (1996), op.cit.

14 Ibid.

15 Silverman, P.R. and Worden, W.J. (2008) 'Children's reactions to the death of a parent', in M.S. Stroebe, R.O. Hansson, H.A.W. Schut and W. Stroebe (eds) *Handbook of Bereavement Research and Practice: 21st Century Perspectives* (pp. 3–26), Washington: APA.

16 Worden (1996), op.cit.

17 Ibid.

18 Ibid.

19 Ibid.

20 Ibid.

21 Gillies, V., Ribbens McCarthy, J. and Holland, J. (2001) *Pulling Together, Pulling Apart: the Family Lives of Young People*, London: Family Policy Studies Centre/Joseph Rowntree Foundation. See also Worden (1996), op. cit.

5 Mourning time: the second year and after

1 Worden (1996), op. cit.

2 Stroebe, Wolfgang and Stroebe, Margaret (1987) *Bereavement and Health*, Cambridge: Cambridge University Press.

3 Worden (1996), op. cit. For children in the Childhood Bereavement Study social problems and changes in self-perception were beginning to surface at 2 years after death. Bereaved children at 2 years had more social problems than non-bereaved children, according both to their parents and their own account. This was more likely in case of dead mother than dead father. Death of parent also affects self-esteem in children although this effect only becomes apparent 2 years after the death. One year after death researchers found no significant differences between bereaved and non-bereaved children on self-esteem, but at 2 years, researchers found 'a large and significant difference between the self-esteem scores of the bereaved and the non-bereaved.' Low self-esteem was associated with more behavioural problems during the first and second year of bereavement. Two years after the death, compared with non-bereaved teens, bereaved teens were more withdrawn, had more anxiety and depression, were more worried about their families, and had more social problems.

4 Williams (2009), op. cit.

5 See Chapter 4, note 4.

6 Fleming, S.J. and Adolph, R. (1986) 'Helping bereaved adolescents: needs and responses', in C.A. Carr and J.N. McNeil (eds) *Adolescence and death*, London: The Hogarth Press, 243–258.

7 McIntyre, Brendan and Hogwood, Jemma (2006) 'Play, Stop and Eject: Creating Film Script Stories with Bereaved Young People', *Bereavement Care* 25(3): 47–49:

In daily life we commonly use narratives to organise and make sense of our experiences and communicate them to others. Telling our stories and the way we tell them, help us to develop a coherent sense of self ... by allowing the individual to gain a new perspective on life events. Similarly it is important to give bereaved children the opportunity to externalise what has happened to them so that they can see themselves separately from their worries and difficulties. This way, the child is not defined by their bereavement, but as a person who had experiences prior to and after the death. It can also relieve some of the emotions connected to the events, such as guilt or blame.

6 Changes and losses: the private kind

1 Little, M., Sandler, I.N., Wolchik, S.A., Tein, J.-Y., and Ayers, T.S. (2009) 'Comparing cognitive, relational and stress mechanisms underlying gender differences in recovery from bereavement-related internalizing problems', *Journal of Clinical Child and Adolescent Psychology* 38(4): 486–500.

2 Worden (1996), op. cit.

3 Ibid.

4 Ibid.

5 Dowdney, (2000), op. cit.

6 Silverman, P.R. and Worden, J.W. (1993) 'Children's reactions to the death of a parent', in W. Stroebe, M. Stroebe and R. O. Hansson, *Handbook of Bereavement: Theory, Research and Intervention*, Cambridge: Cambridge University Press.

7 Worden (1996), op. cit.

8 Brizendine, Louann (2006) *The Female Brain*, New York: Three Rivers Press.

9 Silverman, P.R. and Worden, J.W. (1993) 'Children's reactions to the death of a parent', in W. Stroebe, M. Stroebe and R.O. Hansson, *Handbook of Bereavement: Theory, Research and Intervention*. Cambridge: Cambridge University Press.

10 Williams (2009), op. cit.

11 Ibid.

12 Dowdney, L., Wilson, R., Maugham, B., Allerton, M., Scholfield and Skuse, D. (1999) 'Psychological disturbance and service provision in parentally bereaved children: perspective case-control study', *British Medical Journal* 319: 354–57.

13 Weller, R.A., Weller, E.B., Fristad, M.A., Bowes, J.M. (1991) 'Depression in recently bereaved prepubertal children', *American Journal of Psychiatry* 148: 1526–40.

14 Ibid.

15 Worden (1996), op. cit.

16 Klass, D., Silverman, P.R., and Nickman, S.L. (eds) (1996) *Continuing Bonds: New Understandings of Grief*, Washington, DC: Taylor & Francis.

17 Williams (2009), op. cit.

18 Ibid.

19 Ibid.

20 Ibid.

21 Abdelnoor, Adam and Hollins, Sheila (2004) 'The effects of childhood bereavement on secondary school performance', *Educational Psychology in Practice* 20(1): 43–54.

22 Williams (2009), op. cit.
23 Ibid.
24 Ibid.
25 Ibid.
26 Ibid.
27 Ibid.
28 Ibid.
29 Ibid.
30 Dowdney *et al.* (1999), op. cit. Gersten, J.C., Beals, J. and Kallgren, C.A. (1991) 'Epidemiology and preventive interventions: parental death in childhood as a case example', *American Journal Comm Psychology* 19: 481–500.
31 Sweeting, H., West, P. and Richards, M. (1998) 'Teenage family life, lifestyles and life chances: associations with family structure, conflict with parents and joint family activity', *International Journal of Law, Policy and the Family* 12(1): 15–46.
32 Hankin, B.L., Mermelstein, R. and Roesch, L. (2007) 'Sex differences in adolescent depression: stress exposure and reactivity models', *Child Development* 78: 279–95.
33 Little *et al.* (2009) op. cit.: The researchers found that:

> The loss of a parent during childhood or adolescence presents an extraordinary threat to security of attachment. Bereaved girls' greater propensity to fears of abandonment may reflect their higher emotional sensitivity to loss of an attachment figure, which is likely to potentiate increased sensitivity to threats of interpersonal loss in other social attachments as well as increased likelihood of internalising morbidity.

34 Worden, W.J. and Silverman, P. (2006) in P. Wupperman and C.S. Neumann, 'Depressive symptoms as a function of sex-role, rumination and neuroticism', *Personality and Individual Differences* 40: 189–201.
35 Sandler *et al.* (2010) 'Long term effects of the Family Bereavement Program on multiple indicators of grief in parentally bereaved children and adolescents', *Journal of Consulting and Clinical Psychology* 78(2): 131–43.
36 Hoeksema, N.S. and Morrow, J. (1991) 'A prospective study of depression and its symptoms after a natural disaster: the 1989 Loma Prieta earthquake', *Journal of Personality and Social Psychology* 61: 115–21.
37 Abela, J.R.Z. and Hankin, B.L. (2008) 'Cognitive vulnerability to depression in children and adolescents: a developmental psychopathology perspective', in J. R.Z. Abela and B.L. Hankin (eds) *Handbook of Depression in Children and Adolescents*, New York: Guildford Press, pp. 35–78.
38 Hankin, B.L., Mermelstein, R. and Roesch, L. (2007) 'Sex differences in adolescent depression: stress exposure and reactivity models', *Child Development* 78: 279–95.
39 Tyrka, A.R., Wier, L., Price, L.H., Ross, N., Anderson, G.M., Wilkinson, C.W. and Carpenter, L.L. (2008) 'Childhood parental loss and adult hypothalamic-pituitary-adrenal function', *Biological Psychiatry* 63(12): 1147–54.
40 Kendler *et al.* (2006) 'Towards a comprehensive development model for major depression in men', *American Journal of Psychiatry* 163: 115–24.
41 Tyson-Rawson, K. (1996) 'Relationship and heritage: manifestations of ongoing attachment following father death' in Dennis Klass, Phyllis Silverman and

Steven Nickman (eds) *Continuing Bonds: New Understandings of Grief*, Washington, DC: Taylor & Francis.

42 Williams (2009), op. cit.

43 Ibid.

44 Sandler, I.N., Ma, Y., Tein, J.-Y., Ayers, T.S., Wolchik, S., Keenedy, C. and Mi, R. (2010) 'Long term effects of the Family Bereavement Program on multiple indicators of grief in parentally bereaved children and adolescents', *Journal of Consulting and Clinical Psychology* 78(2): 131–43.

45 Williams (2009), op. cit.

46 Gorrel Barnes *et al.* (1997), op. cit.

47 Worden (1996), op. cit.

7 Changes and losses: the public kind

1. Grossman, Vasily (2010) *The Road*, London: Maclehouse Press, Quercus.
2. For these and other activities, see *Waving Goodbye: An Activities Manual for Children in Grief* (1995) from Dougy Center for Grieving Children, www.dougy.org. Winston's Wish in the UK also have a range of relevant publications and resources, which can be purchased through the Winston's Wish website at www.winstonswish.org.uk.

8 Old grief in new guises

1. Hung, C. Natalie and Rabin, Laura A. (2009) 'Comprehending childhood bereavement by parental suicide: a critical review of research on outcomes, grief process, and interventions', *Death Studies* 33: 781–814.
2. Williams (2009), op. cit.

9 Pathways to the future

1. Williams (2009), op. cit.

BIBLIOGRAPHY

Abdelnoor, Adam, and Hollins, Sheila (2004) 'The effects of childhood bereavement on secondary school performance', *Educational Psychology in Practice* 20(1): 43–54.

Abela, J.R.Z. and Hankin, B. L. (2008) 'Cognitive vulnerability to depression in children and adolescents: a developmental psychopathology perspective', in J.R.Z. Abela and B.L. Hankin (eds) *Handbook of Depression in Children and Adolescents*, New York: Guildford Press, 35–78.

Ajjan, Diana (ed.) (1994) The Day My Father Died, Pennsylvania: Running Press.

Akerman, R. and Statham, J. (2010) Childhood Bereavement Rapid Literature Review, London: Department For Education.

Beauvoir, Simone de (1969) A Very Easy Death, London: Penguin.

Black, D. (1998) 'Coping with loss: bereavement in childhood', *British Medical Journal* 316: 931–33.

Bowlby, J. (2005) *A Secure Base*, London: Routledge.

Braiden, Hannah, McCann, Monica, Barry, Helen and Lindsay, Carrie (2009) 'Piloting a therapeutic residential for children, young people and families bereaved through suicide in Northern Ireland', *Child Care in Practice* 15(2): 81–93.

Brizendine, Louann (2006) *The Female Brain*, New York: Three Rivers Press.

Brown, E. and Goodman R.F. (2005) 'Childhood traumatic grief following September 11 2001: construct development and validation', *Journal of Clinical Child and Adolescent Psychology* 34: 248–59.

Brown, A.C., Sandler, I.N., Tein, J.-Y., Liu, X. and Haine, R.A. (2007) 'Implications of parental suicide and violent death for the promotion of resilience of parentally bereaved children', *Death Studies* 31(4): 301–35.

Brown, E.J., Amaya-Jackson, L., Cohen, J., Handel, S., De Bocanegra, H.T., Zatta, E., Goodman, R.F. and Mannarino, A. (2008) 'Childhood traumatic grief: a multi-site empirical examination of the construct and its correlates', *Death Studies* 32: 899–923.

Casdagli, Penny and Gobey, Francis, with Caroline Griffin (1992) *Grief – the play, writings and workshops*, David Fulton.

Cerel, J., Fristad, M., Weller, E.B. and Weller, R.A. (1999) 'Suicide-bereaved children and adolescents: a controlled longitudinal examination', *Journal of the American Academy of Child and Adolescent Psychiatry* 38: 672–79.

Cerel, J., Fristad, M.A., Weller, E.B. and Weller, R.A. (2000) 'Suicide-bereaved children and adolescents II: parental and family functioning', *Journal of the American Academy of Child and Adolescent Psychiatry* 39: 437–44.

Cheifetz, P.N., Stavrakakis, G. and Lester, E.P. (1989) 'Studies of the affective state in bereaved children', *Canadian Journal of Psychiatry* 34(7): 688–92.

Chick, Sandra, (1989) I Never Told Her I Loved Her, Banbury: Livewire Books.

Cohen, J.A., Mannarino, A.P., Greenberg, T., Padlo, S. and Shipley, C. (2002) 'Childhood traumatic grief: concepts and controversies', *Trauma, Violence, and Abuse* 3(4): 307–27.

Cohen, J.A., Mannarino, A.P. and Staron, V.R. (2006) 'A pilot study of modified cognitive-behavioral therapy for childhood traumatic grief', *Journal of the American Academy of Child and Adolescent Psychiatry* 45: 1465–73.

Crossley, Diana (2000) Muddles, Puddles and Sunshine: Your Activity Book To Help When Someone Has Died (a Winston's Wish publication), Stroud: Hawthorn Press.

Currier, J.M., Holland, J.M. and Neimeyer, R.A. (2007) 'The effectiveness of bereavement interventions with children: a meta-analytic review of controlled outcome research', *Journal of Clinical Child and Adolescent Psychology* 36(2): 253–59.

Doolan, E. (1983) *Counselling Young People*, London: Routledge.

Dougy Center for Grieving Children (1995) *Waving Goodbye: An Activities Manual for Children in Grief*, www.dougy.org.

Dowdney, L., Wilson, R., Maugham, B., Allerton, M., Scholfield and Skuse, D. (1999) 'Psychological disturbance and service provision in parentally bereaved children: perspective case-control study', *British Medical Journal* 319: 354–57.

Dowdney, L. (2000) 'Annotation: childhood bereavement following parental death', *Journal of Child Psychology and Psychiatry* 41(7): 819–30.

Doyle, Derek (1984) Coping with a Dying Relative, Macdonald.

Edelman, Hope (1995) Motherless Daughters: the legacy of loss, London: Hodder and Stoughton.

Fleming, S.J. and Adolph, R. (1986) 'Helping bereaved adolescents: needs and responses', in C.A.Carr and J.N. McNeil (eds) *Adolescence and Death*, London: The Hogarth Press, 243–58.

Gerhardt, Sue (2004) Why Love Matters, London: Routledge.

Gersten, J.C., Beals, J. and Kallgren, C.A. (1991) 'Epidemiology and preventive interventions: parental death in childhood as a case example', *American Journal of Community Psychology* 19: 481–500.

Gillies V., Ribbens McCarthy, J. and Holland, J. (2001) Pulling Together, Pulling Apart: the Family Lives of Young People, London: Family Policy Studies Centre/Joseph Rowntree Foundation.

Golding, Christopher (1991) Bereavement, Marlborough: Crowood Press.

Gorer, G. (1965) *Death, Grief, and Mourning in Contemporary Britain*, London: The Cresset Press.

Gorrel Barnes, J., Thompson, P., Davies, G. and Burchardt, N. (1997) Growing Up in Stepfamilies, Oxford: Oxford University Press.

Grad, O. and Zavasnik, A. (1996) 'Similarities and differences in the process of bereavement after suicide and after traffic fatalities in Slovenia', *Omega* 33: 243–51.

Haine, R.A., Wolchik, S.A., Sandler, I.N. Millsap, R.E. and Ayers, T.S. (2006) 'Positive parenting as a protective resource for parentally bereaved children', *Death Studies* 30(1): 1–28.

Hankin, B.L., Mermelstein, R. and Roesch, L. (2007) 'Sex differences in adolescent depression: stress exposure and reactivity models', *Child Development* 78: 279–95.

Harris, Paul (ed) (2005) *What to Do When Someone Dies*, 9th edition, Consumers' Association and Which? Books.

Hendricks, J., Black, D. and Koplan, T. (1993) When Father Kills Mother: Guiding Children through Trauma and Grief, London: Routledge.

Hodgson Burnett, Frances (1911) The Secret Garden, London: Puffin.

Hoeksema, N.S. and Morrow, J. (1991) 'A prospective study of depression and its symptoms after a natural disaster: the 1989 Loma Prieta earthquake', *Journal of Personality and Social Psychology* 61: 115–21.

Horn, Sandra (1989) Coping with Bereavement, London: Thorsons.

Hung, C. Natalie, and Rabin, Laura A. (2009) 'Comprehending childhood bereavement by parental suicide: a critical review of research on outcomes, grief process, and interventions', *Death Studies* 33: 781–814.

Irish, D.P., Lundquist, K.F. and Nelsen, V.J. (1993) Ethnic Variations in Dying, Death, and Grief: Diversity in Universality, Philadelphia: Taylor & Francis.

Jones, D.R., Goldblatt, P.O. and Leon, D.A. (1984) 'Bereavement and cancer: some results using deaths of spouses from the Longitudinal Study of the Office of Population Census and Surveys', *British Medical Journal* 298: 461–64.

Kaprio, J., Koskenvuo, M. and Rita, H. (1987) 'Mortality after bereavement: a prospective study of 95,647 widowed persons', *American Journal of Public Health* 77: 283–87.

Kendler, K.S., Gardner, C.O. and Prescott, C.A. (2006) 'Towards a comprehensive development model for major depression in men', *American Journal of Psychiatry* 163: 115–24.

Kirwin, K.M. and Hamrin, V. (2005) 'Decreasing the risk of complicated bereavement and future psychiatric disorders in children', *Journal of Child and Adolescent Psychiatric Nursing* 18(2): 62–78.

Klass, D., Silverman, P.R. and Nickman, S.L. (eds) (1996) Continuing Bonds: New Understandings of Grief, Washington, DC: Taylor & Francis.

Kranzler, E.M., Shaffer, D., Wasserman, G. and Davies, M. (1990) 'Early childhood bereavement', *Journal of the American Academy of Child and Adolescent Psychiatry* 29, 513–20.

Krementz, J. (1986) How It Feels When a Parent Dies, London: Gollancz.

Kubler-Ross, Elisabeth (1970) On Death and Dying, London: Tavistock.

Lewis, C.S. (1978) A Grief Observed, London: Faber & Faber.

Lin, K.K., Sandler, I.N., Ayers, T.S., Wolchik, S.A. and Luecken, L.J. (2004) 'Resilience in parentally bereaved children and adolescents seeking protective services', *Journal of Clinical Child and Adolescent Psychology* 33(4): 673–83.

Little, M., Sandler, I.N., Wolchik, S.A., Tein, J.-Y. and Ayers, T.S. (2009) 'Comparing cognitive, relational and stress mechanisms underlying gender differences in recovery from bereavement-related internalizing problems', *Journal of Clinical Child and Adolescent Psychology* 38(4): 486–500.

McCollum, Audrey, T. (1990) The Trauma of Moving, Sage Publications.

McIntyre, Brendan and Hogwood, Jemma, (2006) 'Play, stop and eject: creating film script stories with bereaved young people', *Bereavement Care* 25 (3): 47–49.

McLoughlin, Jane (ed.) (1994) On the Death of a Parent, London: Virago.

Middleton, W., Raphael, B., Martinek, N. and Misso, V. (1993) 'Pathological grief reactions' in W. Stroebe, M. Stroebe, and R.O. Hansson, *Handbook of Bereavement: Theory, Research and Intervention*, Cambridge: Cambridge University Press.

Mitchell, A.M., Wesner, S., Brownson, L., Dysart-Gale, D., Garand, L. and Havill, A. (2006) 'Effective Communication with bereaved child survivors of suicide', *Journal of Child and Adolescent Psychiatric Nursing* 19: 130–36.

Mitchell, A.M., Wesner, S., Garand, L., Gale, D.D., Havill, A. and Brownson, L. (2007) 'A support group intervention for children bereaved by parental suicide', *Journal of Child and Adolescent Psychiatric Nursing* 20: 3–13.

Mundy, Michaelene, (2004) Sad Isn't Bad: A Good-grief Guidebook for Kids Dealing with Loss (Elf-Help Books for Kids), St Meinrad, IN: Abbey Press.

Normand, L. C., Silverman, P.R and Nickman, S.L. Bereaved Children's Changing Relationships with the Deceased in Klass, D., Silverman, P.R. and Nickman S.L. (eds) (1996) *Continuing Bonds: new understandings of grief*. Washington D.C: Taylor & Francis.

Parkes, C.M., Benjamin, B. and Fitzgerald, B.G. (1969) Broken Heart: a statistical study of increased mortality among widowers. *British Medical Journal* 114: 41.

Parkes, Colin Murray (1972) Bereavement, London: Tavistock.

Parkes, Colin Murray and Weiss, Robert S. (1983) Recovery from Bereavement, New York: Basic Books.

Pfeffer, C., Jiang, H., Kakuma, T., Hwang, J. and Metsch, M. (2002) 'Group intervention for children bereaved by the suicide of a relative', *Journal of the American Academy of Child and Adolescent Psychiatry* 41: 505–13.

Pfeffer, C.R., Martins, P., Mann, J., Sunkenberg, M., Ice, A., Danmore, J.P., Gallo, C., Karpenos, I. and Jiang, H. (1997) Child Survivors of Suicide: Psychosocial Characteristics, *Journal of the American Academy of Child & Adolescent Psychiatry*, 36: 1 pp. 65–74.

Pincus, Lily (1976) Death and the Family: The Importance of Mourning, London: Faber & Faber.

Raveis, V.H., Siegel, K. and Karus, D. (1999) 'Children's psychological distress following the death of a parent', *Journal of Youth and Adolescence* 28: 2.

Reed, M.D. (1998) 'Predicting grief symptomatology among the suddenly bereaved', *Suicide and Life-Threatening Behaviour* 21: 385–401.

Romain, Jonathan (1991) Faith and practice: a guide to Reform Judaism today, London: Reform Synagogues of Great Britain.

Rosenblatt, Paul C. (1993) 'Cross-cultural variation in the experience, expression and understanding of grief', in D.P. Irish, K.F. Lundquist and V.J. Nelsen, *Ethnic Variations in Dying, Death, and Grief: Diversity in Universality*, Philadelphia: Taylor & Francis.

Rosenman, L., Shulman, A.D. and Levine, M. (1984) 'Widowed families with children: personal need and societal response', *Institute of Family Studies*, Working Paper No. 7, May.

Rosenman, S. and Rodgers, B. (2004) 'Childhood adversity in an Australian population', *Social Psychiatry and Psychiatric Epidemiology* 39: 695–702.

Rosenman, S. and Rodgers, B. (2006) 'Childhood adversity and adult personality', *Australian and New Zealand Journal of Psychiatry* 40: 482–90.

Rosner, R., Kruse, J. and Hagl, M. (2010) 'A meta-analysis of interventions for bereaved children and adolescents', *Death Studies* 34(2): 99–136.

Rowe, Dorothy (1991) The Courage to Live, London: Fontana.

Saldinger, A., Cain, A. and Porterfield, K. (2003) 'Managing traumatic stress in children anticipating parental death', *Psychiatry* 66(2): 168–81, Summer.

Sandler, I.N., Ayers, T. and Wolchik, S. *et al.* (2003) 'The Family Bereavement Program: efficacy evaluation of a theory-based prevention program for parentally bereaved children and adolescents', *Journal of Consulting and Clinical Psychology* 73(2): 221–28.

Sandler, I.N., Ma, Y., Tein, J.-Y., Ayers, T.S., Wolchik, S., Keenedy, C. and Mi, R. (2010) 'Long term effects of the Family Bereavement Program on multiple indicators of grief in parentally bereaved children and adolescents', *Journal of Consulting and Clinical Psychology* 78(2): 131–43.

Schoen A.A., Burgoyne, M. and Schoen, F.S. (2004) 'Are the developmental needs of children in America adequately addressed during the grief process?' *Journal of Instructional Psychology* 31(2): 143–48.

Scott, Ronald (1991) Coping with Suicide, London: Sheldon Press.

Siegel, K., Masagno, F., Karus, D., Christ, G., Banks, G. and Moynihan, R. (1992) Psychosocial adjustment of children with a terminally ill parent. *Journal of the American Academy of Child/Adolescent Psychiatry*, 31: 327–33.

Siegel, K., Karus, D. and Raveis, V.H. (1996) 'Adjustment of children facing the death of a parent due to cancer', *Journal of the American Academy of Child and Adolescent Psychiatry* 35: 442–50.

Siegel, K., Karus, D., and Raveis, V.H. (1996) 'Patterns of communication with children when a parent has cancer', in L. Baider (ed.) *Cancer and the Family*, New York: John Wiley & Sons, P109–26.

Silberberg, A. (2011) Milo and the Restart Button, London: Simon and Schuster.

Silverman, P.R. (2000) *Never Too Young to Know: Death in Children's Lives*, Oxford: Oxford University Press.

Silverman, P.R. and Worden, J.W. (1993) 'Children's reactions to the death of a parent' in W. Stroebe, M.Stroebe and R.O. Hansson, *Handbook of Bereavement: Theory, Research and Intervention*, Cambridge: Cambridge University Press.

Silverman, P.R. and Worden, W.J. (2008) 'Children's reactions to the death of a parent' in M.S. Stroebe, R.O. Hansson, H.A.W. Schut and W. Stroebe (eds) *Handbook of Bereavement Research and Practice: 21st Century Perspectives*, Washington, D.C.: APA.

Stokes, J.A. and Crossley, D. (2007) As Big As It Gets: Supporting a Child When a Parent is Seriously Ill, Cheltenham: Winston's Wish.

Stokes, J. (2009) The Secret C: Straight Talking About Cancer, Cheltenham: Winston's Wish.

Stroebe, M.S., Hansson, R.O., Schut, H.A.W. and Stroebe, W. (eds) (2008) Handbook of Bereavement Research and Practice: 21st Century Perspectives, Washington, D.C.: APA.

Stroebe, W. and Stroebe, M. (1987) Bereavement and Health, Cambridge: Cambridge University Press.

Stroebe, W. and Stroebe, M. (2008) 'The Mortality of Bereavement', in M.S. Stroebe, R.O. Hansson, H.A.W. Schut and W. Stroebe (eds) *Handbook of Bereavement Research and Practice: 21st Century Perspectives*, Washington, D.C.: APA, 3–26.

Stroebe, W., Stroebe, M. and Hansson, R.O. (1993) Handbook of Bereavement: Theory, Research and Intervention, Cambridge: Cambridge University Press.

Stubbs, D. and Stokes, J. (2008) Beyond the Rough Rock: Supporting a Child Who Has Been Bereaved Through Suicide, Cheltenham: Winston's Wish.

Stubbs, D., Gardner, K. and Nugus, D. (2008) Hope Beyond the Headlines: Supporting a Child Bereaved Through Murder or Manslaughter, Winston's Wish.

Sweeting, H., West, P. and Richards, M. (1998) 'Teenage family life, lifestyles and life chances: associations with family structure, conflict with parents and joint family activity', *International Journal of Law, Policy and the Family* 12(1): 15–46.

Tsuchiya, K. J., Agerbo, E. and Mortensen, P.B. (2005) 'Parental death and bipolar disorder', *Journal of Affective Disorders* 86: 151–59.

Tyrka, A.R., Wier, L., Price, L. H., Ross, N., Anderson, G. M., Wilkinson, C. W. and Carpenter, L.L. (2008) 'Childhood parental loss and adult hypothalamic-pituitary-adrenal function', *Biological Psychiatry* 63(12): 1147–54.

Tyson-Rawson, K. (1996) 'Relationship and heritage: manifestations of ongoing attachment following father death', in Klass, D., Silverman, P., and Nickman S. (eds) *Continuing Bonds: New Understandings of Grief*, Washington, DC: Taylor & Francis.

Van Eerdewegh, M.M., Clayton, P.J. and Van Eerdewegh, P. (1985) 'The bereaved child: variables influencing early psychopathology', *British Journal of Psychiatry* 147, 188–94.

Wallbank, Susan (1991) Facing Grief – Bereavement and the Young, Cambridge: Lutterworth Press.

Walter, Tony (1990) Funerals – and How to Improve Them, London: Hodder & Stoughton.

Waving Goodbye: An Activities Manual for Children in Grief (1995) from Dougy Center, PO Box 86852, Portland, Oregon, OR 97286.

Weller, R.A., Weller, E.B., Fristad, M.A. and Bowes, J.M. (1991) 'Depression in recently bereaved prepubertal children', *American Journal of Psychiatry* 148: 1526–40.

Williams, Caspar (2009) 'Adolescent boys and bereavement: a reflexive and phenomenological-narrative analysis of adult men who lost their fathers in adolescence', MA dissertation, Regent's College London, July.

Willson, Jane Wynne (1989) Funerals Without God: A Practical Guide to Non-religious Funerals, British Humanist Association.

Winn, D. (1987) The Hospice Way, London: Macdonald Optima.

Wood, K., Chase, E. and Aggleton, P. (2006) 'Telling the truth is the best thing: teenage orphans' experiences of parental AIDS-related illness and bereavement in Zimbabwe', *Social Science and Medicine* 63(7): 1923–33.

Worden, J. William (1983) Grief Counselling and Grief Therapy, London: Tavistock.

Worden, J. William (1996) Children and Grief: When a Parent Dies, New York: Guildford Press.

Wupperman, P. and Neumann, C.S. (2006) 'Depressive symptoms as a function of sex-role, rumination and neuroticism', *Personality and Individual Differences* 40: 189–201.

Yule, W. and Canterbury, R. (1994) 'The treatment of post traumatic stress disorder in children and adolescents', *International Review of Psychiatry* 6(2–3): 194–2000.

Zisook, S., Devaul, R.A. and Click, M.A. Jr (1982) 'Measuring symptoms of grief and bereavement', *American Journal of Psychiatry* 139(12): 1590–93.

INDEX